INDIAN USES
OF
NATIVE PLANTS

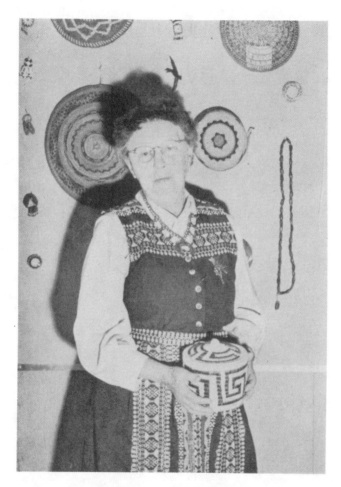

EDITH VAN ALLEN MURPHEY

INDIAN USES
OF
NATIVE PLANTS

Edith Van Allen Murphey

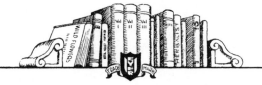

Meyerbooks, *Publisher*
Glenwood, Illinois

Meyerbooks, *Publisher*
P.O. Box 427
Glenwood, Illinois 60425

To Alida C. Bowler

Former Superintendent of Carson Indian Agency
Stewart, Nevada
Who opened the door to the Inter-Mountain Indian world for me

PREFACE

It is with great pride that the Mendocino County Historical Society presents this reprint of *INDIAN USES OF NATIVE PLANTS,* by Edith Van Allen Murphey. We regret that the work was not completed prior to the author's death on August 9, 1968. Mrs. Murphey, who was a charter and honorary life member of the Society, granted the Society permission to reprint her book. All profits realized from the sale of this book will be used for further development of the Mendocino County Museum, 400 East Commerical Street, Willits, California, and the Held-Poage Memorial Home and Research Library, Headquarters of the Mendocino County Historical Society, 603 West Perkins Street, Ukiah, California, 95482.

The Dictionary of Plant Names was edited and corrected to include up-to-date nomenclature. In addition, indexes of Common Names and Scientific Names are included. No other changes have been made in the original text.

Special acknowledgement is due Walter Knight of the East Bay Regional Park District, Oakland, California, for editing the Dictionary of Plant Names and for his valuable work in compiling the Index of Scientific Names. The Index of Common Names was prepared by Laura Keller of the Mendocino County Historical Society.

FOREWORD

In May, 1935, Carson Indian School, Stewart, Nevada, held its first Wild Flower Show. Prizes were offered for the most beautiful specimens, for the most unusual collections and the exhibit that presented the most information about the various ways in which the Indians used the plants.

The various grades in the large boarding school brought in fine collections from the area in their vicinity. Indian Day Schools in other parts of Nevada competed with collections from their areas.

The result was an exceptionally fine flower show, and a demonstration that there existed untapped sources of information about Great Basin plant life, and the uses to which it had been put by its indigenous people.

Interest in the subject was such that new projects were developed that permitted me to serve for ten years in the Inter-Mountain area for United States Bureau of Indian Affairs. Primary interest was in the more practical side: the problem of identifying and eliminating stock-poisoning plants on Indian cattle and sheep ranges.

Contacts made in this phase of the work enabled me to gather data on plant uses in the various tribes.

I should like to express my appreciation to the Paiutes of Pyramid Lake, Walker River and Fort MacDermitt, Nevada, five groups of Shoshones in Nevada, and to Bannocks in Idaho, to the Washoes, to the Utes, and to the Confederated Tribes of Warm Springs, Oregon, and to happy unofficial visits among the Papagos of Arizona, who shared their knoledge of plant uses with me, to the end that unique information should not perish with them, but be preserved for all mankind.

Gratitude is also rendered to all United States Indian Service officials and their families, especially to Alida C. Bowler, former Superintendent of Carson Indian Agency, and to all Forestry officials and their personnel.

State universities which aided in plant identifications in the States of Nevada, Wyoming, Utah, to Oregon, Oregon State College at Corvallis, Oregon, Idaho and Montana gave valuable assistance through their Botany Departments.

My cousins, Van Allen and Jesusita Lyman of Costa Rica helped materially in the publication of this book; also my cousin, Mrs. Charles Leslie Mitchell of San Antonio, Texas.

The line drawing of plants are by Mrs. Ella M. Hanks.

INTRODUCTION

This work is founded on work done on stock poisoning plants for U.S. Indian Service over a period of ten years, chiefly in the Rocky Mountain area, and over fifty years' residence in Mendocino County, California, which has a large Indian population.

A brief winter visit to Papago Reservation, Sells, Arizona, 1948, was most instructive. These were experiences based on personal observation, not a matter of official record.

Botanical identifications were furnished in most instances from the State University nearest the Reservation where work was being done. Especial thanks are due to Oregon State College at Corvallis, Oregon, which made identifications regardless of my location. Pressed specimens were sent each university to add to its herbarium, frequently from areas never before cruised by botanists.

Besides Oregon State College, University of Wyoming, Utah State Agricultural College, Brigham Young University, University of Nevada, and University of California were most helpful.

Work done on stock poisoning plants began at Carson Indian Agency at Stewart, Nevada, when drouth cattle issued to Indians from Dust Bowl areas, began eating all plants they found, and died in consequence.

Up to this time, Nevada Indians had very little stock, nor hardly any horses, so a survey became necessary, and under guidance of Supt. Alida Bowler continued for five growing seasons, with a library of pressed specimens' scrap books of full information and constant field work. These Indians had hitherto learned about poisonous plants by trial and error—those poisonous to human beings. They knew about a very few: Death Camas, which defeated its own purpose, by being emetic, poison hemlock or parsnip, well known to them as a suicide root, and the Buffalo flower or golden pea, seeds sometimes eaten by little children, with vomiting and purging consequences.

A delightful side-line, in connection with the investigation of the Indians' knowledge of stock poisoning plants, was the discovery of medicinal uses of plants, and other uses followed as a matter of course.

Foods from native plants, and migrations which were seasonal harvests of bulbs, roots and seeds fitted in at times when meat was hard to get.

At first, it was difficult to secure information about native uses, but when it was made plain that it was desirable that the knowledge possessed by them should not be lost, but made a matter of record they cooperated willingly and proudly.

Especially were the Shoshones plant conscious. More than any other groups had they studied plant families, and had a rough botany of their own.

Especial appreciation is due Miss Alida C. Bowler, former Supt. of Carson Indian Agency, whose constant backing helped establish the live-stock business firmly in Indian areas in Nevada, and in compiling this present record of Indian uses of native plants, to Prof. E. F. Castetter of University of New Mexico, who by correspondence and by sending me his bulletins, showed me the best way to present the knowledge collected from my friends, the Indians.

My gratitude to all Indians who have helped in this history. This record is theirs, and will keep their tribal names alive forever.

Lastly, to my co-workers in Indian Service, I express my pleasant memory of their constant helpfulness and cooperation.

To all, I thank you.

Sincerely,

EDITH V. A. MURPHEY

CONTENTS

BASKETRY - - - - - - 1

INDIAN FOODS - - - - - - 12

FAMINE FOODS - - - - - 16

BEVERAGES - - - - - - 17

FEASTS - - - - - - 18

GREENS - - - - - - 23

MEAT - - - - - - 23

NUTS - - - - - - - 24

SEEDS - - - - - - 26

THE SALT JOURNEY - - - - - 29

MEDICINAL PLANTS - - - - 36

CEREMONIALS AND MAGIC - - - 50

BOWS AND ARROWS - - - - - 51

DYE PLANTS - - - - - - 53

TANNING HIDES - - - - - 55

ODDS AND ENDS - - - - - 55

HAIR - - - - - - 57

TEPEES - - - - - - 58

TOBACCO - - - - - - 60

DICTIONARY - - - - - - 63

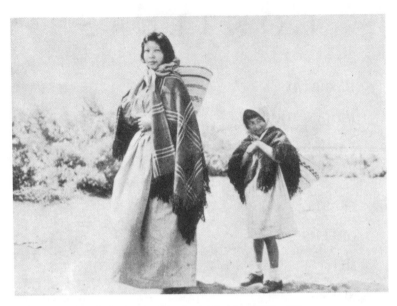

Seed Gathering Basket worn by Paiute Women

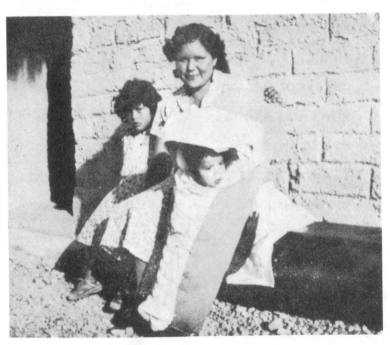

Death Valley Baby Basket

BASKETRY

This subject will be treated by States. Because the writer has spent more time in California and Nevada, and because they join borders, they will be taken up, beginning at the northern boundary of California and proceeding South.

An Indian legend is as follows: "The world was all water, and Saghalee Tyee, (Great Chief) was above it. He threw up out of the water at shallow places large quantities of mud, and that made land. He made trees to grow, and he made Man out of mud, and instructed him in what he should do. When the man grew lonesome, he made a woman for his companion, and taught her to tan hides, to gather berries, and how to find roots. . . . Woman slept and dreaming of how she could please her husband she prayed to Saghalee Tyee to help her. He breathed on her, and gave her something that she could not see, or hear, or smell or touch. It was in a little basket, and by it, all the arts of design and skilled handicraft were given to her descendants."

Basketry is one of the most ancient of arts. On the Northwest Coast, it undoubtedly preceded pottery. This was due perhaps to the great wealth of material right at hand.

Along the Trinity and Klamath rivers in northwest California and on the high ridges sloping down to Hoopa Valley the shrubs and colorants so valuable were many and abundant.

HOOPA BASKETRY

Primitive man needs first of all something to sustain life—food. Food needs something to gather it in, something in which to prepare it, something to cook it in, something to store it in—hence, Baskets.

Beginning literally on the ground, containers for food were made. These varied in size and shape with their use. A conical open work basket served equally well for carrying wood or fish. They were usually woven of willow, and bound with grapevine. A more closely woven shape served for acorns and the many kinds of grass seeds or berries.

The burden or pack basket was formerly carried by a sort of tump line or pack strap, and a forehead pad accompanied it. Nowadays the pack strap comes across the shoulders and the head is put through. Companion to the seed basket was the seed beater. This was a wicker disk with a long handle. Holding the burden basket in the left hand, the seed seeker had only to stoop slightly to beat the ripe seed into her basket, beater held in her right hand.

In picking up acorns, if they were abundant, the woman left the basket on her back, and squatting down, threw them over her head into the basket.

After gathering seeds came the winnowing process to clean all dirt and chaff away from them. Winnowing baskets had wide shallow shapes, rather pyramidal, deeper than they looked which made the heavy seed pile up in the botton. They were closely woven, so that even tiny seeds could not go through and be wasted. Material for these was usually hazel for the rods, and redbud bark for the patterns. A favorite pattern was the quail topknot.

Wind was a great help in cleaning seeds. The right kind of a day was usually chosen, and neighbors worked together very comfortably. Sometimes when seeds were under-ripe or had been stunted, the husks would stick fast, and seed would not clean satisfactorily. Under such circumstances an old basket was used, and hot ashes were placed in it. Then the seeds were put in, tossed around, and tossed again. Heat made the husks fly off, and wind took them away. Heat also gave the seeds a toasted flavor.

Meal made from seeds was called pinole. It was usually eaten raw out of a small basket.

Hazel brush was used for sieves of various degrees of fineness; some were fine as flour sieves. They frequently had fancy borders with a hem-stitched effect.

After the seeds had been cleaned, they were pounded to meal on a flat stone, on which was placed a mortar basket, which kept the seeds from scattering or being blown away by the wind. The pestle was of stone larger at top than at bottom. Sometimes a handhold was nicked at the top. The mortar basket was usually an old pack basket, with its point cut off. The worker sat on the ground with her legs over either side of the basket, holding it firmly.

The foundation of heavy closely woven baskets was split roots of cedar, spruce, Digger pine or other conifers. Besides burden baskets many round cooking baskets, called "acorn soup baskets" were made. Originally these were intended to cook in with hot stones. After the mush was prepared, hot stones were dropped in and they really cooked, too. These baskets varied in size, some being really storage baskets, and some were just right for individual soup bowls. It is unlikely that anyone cooks in baskets nowadays, but the name persists.

The smaller the basket, the more likely that it would have a border pattern of *Xerophyllum tenax,* or Basket grass. This is originally bleached to a silvery tone, but with age it becomes golden. Usually the pattern does not show through on the inside.

A favorite pattern for a burden basket was the "V" of wild geese flying. Many patterns become changed over the years, but the Wild Goose pattern complete with "V" and flying scout outriders, is plainly recognizable.

Waste baskets, market baskets, whose shapes show plainly the white influence which finds them so convenient, are made of willow and occasionally sarvis or service berry juice gives a black dye, used in stripes. Native name for this is "Makoolth."

Baby baskets are made of various materials, willow, hazel and osier dogwood. They are slipper shaped, and have a little seat in them. The top runs up to a loop-like handle, which sometimes serves to support another basket, inverted to make a shade. In Mendocino County the Indian men make such baby baskets as are still used of narrow-leaved or silver willow. Blankets are placed on the basket, tucked around the baby, who sleeps sitting up, sometimes a pillow or diapers are put under him to make the bed soft, and then a buckskin string is laced crosswide through opposite loops to hold the baby firmly. Balance of blanket's outside is gathered and tucked around his feet in a closed bunch, and the string secures it. Hoopa name for this basket is "Lox-too."

BASKET PLANTS

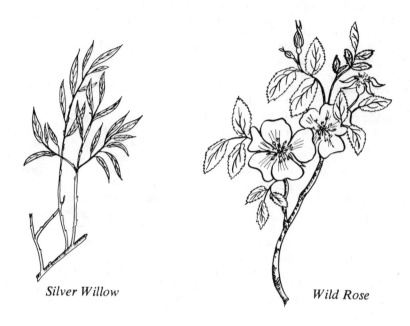

Silver Willow

Wild Rose

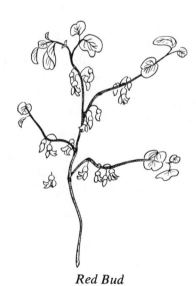

Red Bud

These baskets are carried on the back. There is much to be said for their convenience and the child's comfort and security. The child's back is supported at all times, and with a piece of mosquito netting to keep out flies, plenty of fresh air is obtained.

Hoopa trinket baskets are usually made with a foundation of very finely cut spruce roots, with an overlay of Basket grass. Patterns are sometimes brightly colored. The cream colored, occasionally pale green of the Basket grass covers all the outside of the basket, except at the very bottom where the basket began. This is sometimes a round of roots.

Basket grass is sometimes dyed with alder bark in a brilliant burnt orange shade, which fades with age to a rich brown. The bark, usually the inner or second bark, is cut up into inch pieces and cooked until soft. Then it is chewed and chewed and chewed by the weaver until all the dye is chewed out of it. This dye-juice is ejected from the mouth into a soapstone dish, usually rectangular, rather shallow, and the grass is soaked in this dye, and used as needed. Acid in the saliva is the mordant that sets the color.

On Hoopa Reservation, Five Finger maiden hair fern grows to an unbelievable height. This has a polished brilliantly black stem, which is used to good advantage in patterns, despite its seeming fragility.

A giant fern, *Woodwardia radicans,* grows in graceful profusion. In the mid-rib or backbone of the huge fronds of this fern are to be found two fibers suitable for basketry. These are stripped and handled much as lengths of yarn would be. They are dyed with alder, and sometimes with Wolf Moss.

Wolf Moss is a yellow-green lichen which grows on pine and fir trees it gives a canary yellow, which requires nothing to set the color. This is Evernia vulpina.

Alder and Wolf Moss are seldom used on the same basket.

Porcupine quills are frequently dyed with Wolf Moss. They are chiefly used on the basket hats or Squaw Caps, which are now rarely seen. These caps are exceedingly fine and well-fitting. Only widows wore them, foundation of spruce roots, pattern of maiden hair fern stems or of alder bark dyed basket grass, or of quills, usually yellow. Formerly, as a sign of grief, before knives and scissors were used, the hair was burned off at the neckline. Then pine pitch was smeared on the hair and the "Squaw cap" put on. This was worn for one year, without combing.

A characteristic basket, not common elsewhere, is the basket used for tobacco. Small and round, perfect in shape as a baby's cheek it is of the same fine weave as the trinket baskets. The basket comes up to small opening at the top. A flat cover is woven which matches in pattern the rest of the basket. This cover has a buckskin string laced to loops on the top of the basket. The spruce roots of the basket keep the tobacco from drying out and the cover excludes the air. Appropriately the Smoker family makes the best tobacco baskets.

Great ceremonial dances are still held in northern California, particularly among the Yurok, Karok and Hoopa Indians. The Jump Dance is one in which treasures of regalia and obsidian knives are displayed. Especially handsome are baskets which contain the great obsidian knives and ornaments of the dance. These are held in the hands of the dancers. They are in shape like a music roll, and are of the same weave as the tobacco baskets, but are heavier. Patterns are usually in black of the five-finger fern, overlay of basket grass, foundation of spruce roots.

Head-dresses for Jump Dance have foundation of white deerskin, and broad bands of redheaded woodpecker scalps, bordered by the iridescence of humming birds' feathers, are worn on the head, usually these are in diamond shaped patterns, and are strikingly beautiful.

Traveling south from Hoopa Reservation there is another Reservation called Round Valley Reservation, where remnants of seven tribes still live. The original inhabitants of this beautiful valley were called Yukis. The mountains originally were occupied by Wailakis, and five other tribes were brought in as to a concentration camp in the days of President Fillmore from the Mother Lode. These other tribes were Concow, Numlaki, Pit River, Pomo, and Eel River Indians.

No basket makers are left in Round Valley now, but further south in Mendocino and Lake Counties, Pomo is the dominant basketry. In all of North America, there is no more cosmopolitan basketry, using both twined and coiled ware in every variety. Abundance of good materials is partly responsible for this, also that the Pomos were an amiable peace-loving people with plenty of natural food at their door, so they did not have to wander needlessly, and had no energy wasted by war.

YUKI BASKETRY

On the Round Valley Reservation, the original inhabitants were Yukis. Materials were much the same as those used by their neighbors, except that in addition to those, Yukis used maple and honeysuckle. The natural shrubs, dogwood, the small flowered kind, the redbud and digger pine they used too.

Patterns were simple, the commonest was a series of bands in color each one course in width, when the two ends met, there was a little step so that Row 2 was just a jog higher than Row 1. Sometimes a gap was left. This frequently is a means of identification. Also Yuki work runs from right to left, as one faces the basket. Pomo runs from left to right.

Grapevine was also freely used in mortar baskets and burden twined baskets. They made coarse sifters for buckeye meal, and made seedbeaters. Use of feathers for decoration borrowed from Pomos.

WAILAKI OR WYLACKIE BASKETS

These were people to the north of Round Valley, the mountaineers. They used digger pine roots, basket grass for overlay in burden baskets and in acorn soup baskets, these were cooking bowls, hot stones use. For mortar baskets, and heavy storage baskets, grapevine bound the stiff hoops which formed the upper edge. Sifters were usually of hazel.

Pine and fir roots were laid in hot ashes, and split down fine. Their patterns were those of earth and sky. Wild Goose flight was a favorite. Practically no trinket or ceremonial baskets. Carrying straps were of buckskin or rawhide.

Concow baskets were formerly made in Round Valley, they borrowed freely from their neighbors for patterns and shapes, especially from the Pomos. No baskets made in Round Valley now.

POMO BASKETS

The rich soil supported numbers of willows, sedges and ferns and shrubs and their preparation was an art in itself.

WILLOW (*Salix sessilifolia*) common along the rivers was considered best for certain types of basketry, it could be split very fine for "Boms," or foundation rods. Hazel brush, (*Corylus californica*), was much desired by those living close to foothills, slender stems used for sieves, fish traps and warp for sedge baskets. Redbud (*Cercis canadensis*), is used variously as foundation, as sewing material in coiled baskets. This is called "Millay." The bark is peeled for red-brown for pattern. The inside wood is white.

Root baskets are made from roots of a sedge (*Carex Mendocinoensis*), Pomo name, "Kahoom," or water-gift. These long roots sometimes reach five or six feet in length. They are soaked overnight in water, and the weaver, peels off the bark or outer skin, and rolls it in small coils. The remaining root can be split into many strands, used as "Boms," for foundation. There are sedges, called blackroot sedge, which have a central section, coal-black, which color can be deepened by burying in manure or in blue mud. The botanical name is *Scirpus maritimus* and Indian name is "Tsu-wish." It is brittle and cranky, but the color is good, especially if blackened with fresh juice of poison oak (*Rhus diversiloba*). Also for fern root, the same method is used. Rusty iron or oakbark infusion will change redbud bark from rust color to black.

Fish traps, seed beaters and openwork burden baskets are frequently made by the men from Digger pine, fir or grapevine in the simplest form of weaving. These are from the roots of the conifers, which are heated in warm ashes for awhile. This not only seasons them, but renders them more pliable. Small woody parts of wild grapevine, which are flexible are used for the margin of large burden baskets.

Mortar baskets are also made from fir roots, but frequently an old pack basket has its point and bottom cut off at the right height to fit the pounding rock.

Besides the heavier baskets Pomo men formerly made baby baskets of willow or hazel.

For the finer baskets, nutmeg roots (*Tumion Californica*) "Kobi," were sometimes made into splints, but usually "Kah-hoom," water gift, was favored, the outer covering being made into thread for pattern. Like the Hoopas, the Pomos had their ceremonial baskets, boat baskets, they called them, quite long, 12 to 15 inches, with blunt rounded ends, four ot 6 inches deep or larger, curving in at the top. These were the containers for ceremonial feathers, yellow-hammer headbands, head ornaments, etc. These could be in either one-stick or three-stick weave.

Trinket baskets could be any size, but usually the finer the weave the smaller the basket. Feather baskets were sometimes entirely covered with feathers. These were usually the green heads of mallards, or the red scalps of woodpeckers punctuated rows alternating occasionally with small white beads. The red feathers were not woven solidly as the duck feathers were, but were placed singly. Sometimes yellow from breast of larks marked a zigzag pattern on the green. Frequently the upper margin of a basket bore quail plumes, and again Indian money made of clamshell would be sewed solidly along the top edge of a basket. When feathers were used, pains were taken to place them in the same manner as they lay on the bird.

Besides the one-stick, a continuous coil, and three-stick, roughly analogous to treble crochet, there are heavy weaves, rarely made now called "Tee" and "Bam-tush," these are really double baskets intended for hard use and storage purposes. There was another weave called "Shu-set," no longer made, which was superbly carried out in burden baskets and in occasional trinket baskets.

The improvements and cultivations of civilization have literally up rooted many of the best sources of basket material for the Pomos. Many of the younger generations find preparation of materials so hard to find, too tedious to work with, and care little about patterns handed down by word of mouth to their mothers and grandmothers, but it is pleasant to know that just out of Ukiah, the County-seat of Mendocino County, there is a small Indian village called Pinoleville. Formerly there was an Indian school there, but now the children go by bus to Ukiah, and the former schoolhouse was given by Indian Service to the Pomo Women's Club, who stand for all that makes for improvement of their members and their families.

Among their projects is the perpetuation of the art of basketry. Some expert weavers and their daughters continue to make baskets, and continually have a back-log of orders ahead, from museums and collectors. Mrs. Annie Burke, an octogenarian, and her daughter, Mrs. Elsie Allen weave constantly and keep alive all that is best and beautiful in this native art. There are other members of this club who are equal in their interest and industry. Lake County women have many weavers, and some of them, all Pomos, also belong to this club.

Baby Baskets. Made by the men, of heavy willow sticks, sometimes of hazel, in an "U" shape. The child sits in the bottom of the "U," with its blankets around and under it, laced in by buckskin thongs crisscrossed through side loops on the basket sides. A heavy piece of wood comes at the top and a bit of mosquito bar, or muslin may be draped over it, to keep sun and insects away from the baby. Some tribes use a small flat basket fastened at the top for a shade. The Pomo name for this cradle basket is "Sekah."

DEATH VALLEY SHOSHONE BASKETRY

These Indians, while in California, are allied to the Nevada Indians. During the winter of 1939-40, the writer was in charge of a small trading post at Furnace Creek on Death Valley Monument, where the remnant of a tribe, mostly women, makes fine baskets.

These are Panamint Shoshones, and their materials are decidedly of the desert variety. For the foundation of all baskets, a willow growing at fairly high elevations is used. This is *Salix lasiandra*. This is gathered before it has sprouted leaves, and is peeled before it is too dry. The bark or peeling is carefully saved and made into small coils, which are used as thread to wind about the coiled switches. All material is kept damp as it is used.

For pattern, a very handsome black is procured from a desert plant known as Devil horn or Unicorn plant, Martynia proboscides. "Muzzatacion." This plant has a trailing stem, the seedpod is like a long limber chilipepper pod. When it is ripe and dry, it is deep black. These dry pods are carefully saved and shredded. In some places for the convenience of the basket makers this plant is cultivated. If not black enough, the pieces may be buried in wood ashes, to deepen the shade.

A fine red is procured from freshly dug roots of the Joshua tree, *Yucca brevifolia*. This red is the natural color. If black is needed, it may be obtained from the same source. A slow fire is built on top of the ground directly above the roots for three days. When this has been done, the tree is pulled over by a rope, gently, so as not to break the roots. The roots will be of an unfading black. The name for this pattern material, red or black is "Oomp."

For very fine baskets, the root of a sedge is used. This is *Carex ex-siccata,* or Tall swamp sedge. Indian name: "Matso-zump." The root is buried in still warm ashes, with water added. This makes a fine black.

A brown that shades imperceptibly into green is used by these Indians and by Mission Indians too. This is obtained from the stems of wire grass, *Juncus Mexicanus,* or it may be Balticus.

Deer grass, *Epicampes rigens*—for which no local name was obtained— is used as thread, very white, very long, and very fine.

Occasionally a dusty pink appears in blocks or petal shapes in these baskets. Usually these are the ones which have bird patterns on them. These bright bits of color are bits of feathers from the red-shafted flicker, or yellow-hammer, woven in just as grass would be. One may always be sure of the ancestry of the baskets bearing these marks. Only a few women know this technique, and they are all of one clan, tracing back to the tiny hamlet of Darwin, California.

Basket shapes show desert influence. To avoid evaporation, or keep out heat, in many places, in early days, baskets were small and flat on the bottom. They tapered widely upward to broad and graceful shoulders swelling gently into a cuff or bottleneck. Such a basket is called "Pono." The best trinket baskets are frequently made in this shape.

Flat-bottomed bowls, small at the base, with straight sides flaring up to a wide top, are extremely decorative and useful. These are usually the work of one woman who confines herself entirely to copying the "rock-writings" so common in the Southwest. They are all black and white, and are called "Ong-mo." About ten inches across the top.

Occasionally a boat basket, long, with rounded ends, is made. In Northern California this shape was reserved for ceremonial baskets, to contain feathers, etc., used in dances. This is in a three-stick weave, three rows worked on at once, like treble crochet. Patterns used on this style, here, usually of animals.

Mountain sheep, with proudly curling horns, lizards, birds and butterflies all are popular designs for basketry.

Probably the chacuala lizard and the butterfly are the most popular designs. To one who knows the hardships which have been endured by these mature women, there is a degree of pathos in the persistency and delicacy with which they etch the butterfly, most ethereal and ephemeral of all the denizens of the desert, on their baskets, as if seeking to hold permanently the beauty which so lightly flits by their very practical lives.

In the possession of National Park Service is an ancient basket waterbottle. This was buried in a sandstorm in Johnson Canyon, nearly a hundred years ago, and was unearthed in 1939.

When found, it had many pine-nuts stored in it. Its shape was still graceful, and it was only broken at the narrow neck, where the great weight of sand had cracked it. It had originally been pitched with pine gum, inside and out, and bright bits of resin still trickled from it. When new, it must have held more than two gallons of water. When the finder, took it home to his wife, she at once remembered that her father's oldest sister was said to have tried to make the largest waterbottle anywhere around, and this was undoubtedly it.

PAPAGO BASKETRY

It was the writer's good fortune to spend two months at Santa Rosa Village out from Sells Agency, southeast from Phoenix, Arizona, a few years ago. Throughout this Agency there are many scattering villages of Papago Indians, related to the Pimas, but with quite different basketry.

These villages seldom have a population of more than 200 souls. It is "not considered good for people to live too thick," so like most desert communities they follow the water. There is a large underground river in this part of Arizona, and when the Government gets a well, the village is built around it, locating first the church.

There is usually a government school, and its kitchen and workrooms are useful to the older women who bring sewing, and occasionally their basket material to prepare. All over their desert country are the plants which furnish them foundation and color for their baskets. The weaving is different, but the plants are much the same as those used by the Panamint Shoshones, and the Moapa and other Nevada Indians.

On the high plains they find Bear grass (*Nolina Bigelovii*), also called Basket grass, and gather it late in Spring. This is bleached or used in the green color, as the weaver prefers, then in summer the women go to some section where the yucca is plentiful. They cut the youngest leaves from the yucca's crown, and split them down to the same size, when they are laid to bleach in the sun.

Never a dull moment in the basket maker's life. In Fall when the pods of Devil horn, or "E-hook," as the Papagos call it, are ripe, they too are gathered. These pods have long sharp hooks extending out from the pod proper, and as they dry they split off, so that each piece furnishes at least two good pieces. These are buried in damp ground to set the color and make them more pliable. When the weaver is ready to make her basket, all material is handled damp.

There is a great deal to be said for Papago basketry. All hands work at this art, young as well as old, tirelessly, and with a keen enjoyment of competition, both in fineness of work, and in looking up old patterns and those with a story behind them.

A trip to Sells from Santa Rosa village in the school bus going to the Agency for supplies, revealed that this was going to be Basket Day at Covered Wells, and other spots along the way. Many passengers were on the bus, each with flour-sack or two with baskets inside, to sell or exchange at the trading posts. Some had large baskets, these were orders, and were carefully covered from view. Young weavers were shy about showing their work, but were commended by the older women, and sometimes with a word about materials, the product of experience.

Trays found useful by whites for fruit or other uses, were common, some had little handles at the ends. Practically all were black and white, except those which had green yucca used in the large plaques which are used as pictures to hang on the wall. A favorite design was "Itoi's House." Itoi is Elder Brother, and his house is identifiable with what the books call the Pima maze. A large circular plaque, fifteen inches in diameter, has a loop at top to hang it by. From the center rays stretch out, ever growing larger until they reach the margin. In the foreground stands "Itoi" with outstretched arms. The person examining the plaque selects a ray, which is green, foundation white—and traces its progress around the plaque until it reaches the center. If the journey is too soon terminated, it is unfavorable, but "Itoi's" house has many mansions, and usually the finish is satisfactory.

Some interesting plaques bore a clan mark, a turtle, or a hawk with lizard hanging from his bill. These were family affairs, a gift of one of these indicated deep friendship.

The basket makers are very suggestible. Having asked about a small basket to hold short stemmed flowers, such as violets, a pretty one was produced with upstanding handles. When asked what name to ask for if a repeat order should be forthcoming, the sober answer was: "With ears."

Baskets of a work basket type had covers, with a flange which effectually made them sand and dust-tight, and sold very reasonably. Foundation of cat-tail or grass stems. For black of "E-Hook," see Death Valley Shoshones, preparation of Devil horn, and for black of Joshua tree, the same. Preparation is identical.

OREGON BASKETS

With very little basket experience in Oregon, little was learned about baskets; such as were seen on Warm Springs Reservation were old huckleberry baskets, not made there, in soft weaves. Those seen at Root Feasts were probably made by Klickitats. They were tied in front of the huckleberry picker, and berries stripped into them. Inside and foundation of split roots of cedar, ornamentation of golden squaw grass.

Yellow dye was made from Oregon grape, red brown from second alder bark, black from strands colored with acorns or oak soaked in mud.

SALLY BAGS: CORNHUSK BAGS

Sally Bags were formerly made by the Wasco Indians, an art borrowed from Nez Perce Indians who were horse Indians. These soft bags were originally saddle bags. Foundation of Indian hemp or any of the native milkweeds. Bottoms and top margins were of woven cedar bark.

Corn was introduced to the Nez Perces by missionaries. This new material cornhusk was eagerly seized by the weavers, it was fascinating in its possibilities, flexible and easy to dye with native dyes, rose from madder roots or berries, green from juniper and sage, burnt orange from alder bark.

Some bags had strips of dyed cornhusks in patterns, overlaying not showing on the inside of the bag; another bag overlaying and twining to show through on the inside.

Baby baskets, not now much used, were called "Tum-tsuss-iss." Osier dogwood, "Lotzanee' and willow, "Ae light 'k." materials used.

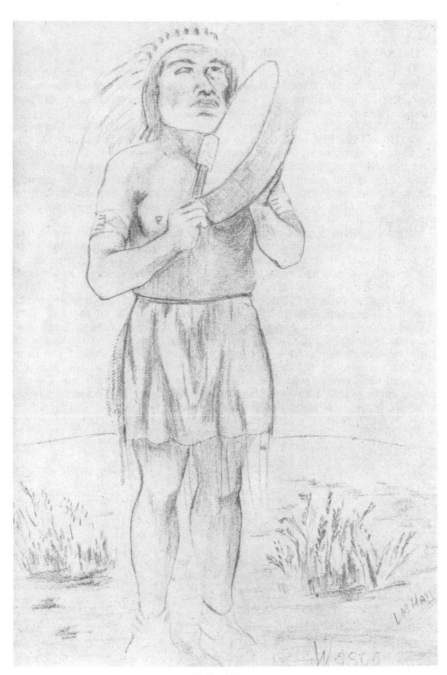

Call to Feast

INDIAN FOODS

BULBS AND ROOTS

Many Indian tribes were called Digger Indians. This was because much of their food was obtained by digging bulbs and roots. Digging was usually done after a plant had ripened seed. Bulbs dug then would keep till used; if dug too green, they would spoil.

BISCUIT-ROOT, Indian name, "Cous." Botanical name, *Cogswellia Cous.* One of the first food-roots to come to white men's attention was this Biscuit-root. Sacajawea, Indian woman guide of Lewis and Clark, showed them this interesting plant, also how to cook it. The leaves grow but a short distance above the ground, the flower is small and white or pale lavender. The root grows in a peculiar fashion, one small round root above another, usually about three, size of golf balls, becoming smaller as they go deeper into the ground.

Oregon Indians have a ceremony in connection with these roots. They are eaten at the first feast of the new year. Roots must not be dug before the seed is ripe. If dug too green they taste something like turpentine. A stew is made of fish and roots are added. Meat stew is made in the same way, but meat and fish are never mixed.

This feast is called the Root Feast. It is held in the Long House, usually built in an abandoned sawmill. All the chiefs are seated at the end of the hall. All are dressed in handsome beaded buckskin costumes. Each chief has a small drum of hide stretched over a ring. There is no bottom to the drum, rawhide thongs stretch the drum and furnish a hand-hold. The drum, plate size, is held by the left hand, even with the ear. The one drumstick is padded and covered with buckskin. The drum is not struck but the stick gives a rubbing roll, continuing from one to another. The Head Chief sings as he drums, and calls upon them, one by one to join in the singing.

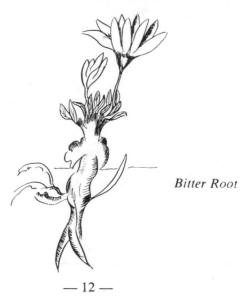

Bitter Root

While this is going on, women in colorful beaded buckskin robes bring in strips of new straw matting—this used to be mats made of tules—which are laid down in front of the guests. Plates of enamel and spoons are set down, and extras such as oranges, and cup-cakes are put at each place.

When the singing is concluded women bearing platters of roots and fish appear in processional. Other foods are carried, and in quick succession each plate receives its quota. When all is in readiness the chiefs come down from their raised seats, and take their places before the food with a final chant of thanksgiving.

BITTER-ROOT, Botanical name: *Lewisia rediviva.* Indian names: "Ax six sixie," Blackfeet; "Kanigda," Yerington Paiutes; "Pe ah ke." Warm Springs, Oregon; "Gunga," Shoshone, Smoky Valley, Nevada.

Bitter-Root, which belongs to the portulaca family, has a very lovely flower, of a deep rose color. After the flower drops its petals, the papery calyx remains with tiny black seeds. The seeker for roots can follow these ghost flowers about, and dig numbers of roots. The roots are like a forked radish, with bitter covering. The roots are thrown into water to soak off the bitter bark, then after drying they are ready for the feast kettle. The taste is like rice, with a bitter after-taste. When dried for winter use, they are called macaroni-root. A grain sack full of cleaned roots was once considered a fair exchange for a good horse.

At wedding feasts in Oregon the bride's relatives came bringing gifts of corn-husk or Sally-bags filled with Biscuit-root, Bitter-root and Camas bulbs for the young folks to start housekeeping with. The groom's relatives contributed parfleches of dried meat and sometimes, blankets or furs.

ARROWHEAD. TULE POTATO. Botanical name: *Sagittaria latifolia.* Indian names: "Wapato," Oregon; "Katniss," Algonquin.

This is an aquatic plant with a tuberous root. A species of this plant grows in China. Chinese in lower Sacramento Valley, California eat it freely. Lewis and Clark found it at the mouth of the Willamette and considered it equal to the potato, and valuable for trade. Indian women collected it in shallow water from a canoe, separating the bulb from the root with their toes. The roots were boiled or roasted in the ashes, and used with fish or meat.

BREADROOT, INDIAN OR PRAIRIE APPLE. Botanical name: *Psoralea esculenta,* also called Indian Turnip, French name: Pomme blanche, or Pomme de Prairie. Indian name: "Tipsinnah," Sioux.

This plant grows on high plains from Manitoba west to the Rockies. It was gathered before the tops died down, and bunches were braided together and hung up for winter use. The roots were boiled or roasted or dried and ground into meal for in soups. It was in high favor with early travelers in Indian country and with trappers, also Indians. John Colter of Lewis and Clark's expedition, escaped from the Indians and lived for a month on this and an edible thistle.

BRODIAEAS and CALOCHORTUS. These small bulbs are abundant in northern California, and were variously known as Indian onion, though not of that family—and as Indian potatoes. They were dug with a digging stick, usually made from mountain mahogany. The seeds of brodiaeas, small and black were put into pinole. The flowers were beautifully marked and colored, and as the bulbs grew in beds, they were easily harvested.

For seasoning, wild onions and garlic were used. The little onion which grows on sand bars in quantity used to be barbecued. The tall pink flowered one which grows in wet meadows is used in soup and stews. This called "Gink" in Shoshone, "Papusi" in Paiute and "Bostick" in Washoe. The little one is called "Sham am way" in Oregon. "When the onion blooms, the salmon run." That is when the Warm Springs Indians go to Celilo to fish.

GARLIC, Botanical name, *Allium falcifolium*. Indian name: "Padzimo," Shoshone.

In the high mountains on dry rocky plains grows a dwarf pink garlic. It has blue-green sickle-shaped leaves, flat, and a pretty flower. The bulb is also deep pink color and is very strong in taste.

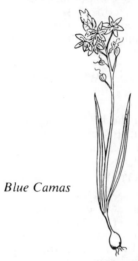

Blue Camas

CAMAS, Botanical name: *Camassia esculenta*. Indian name "Ketten," Wailaki (Calif.); "Kogi," Paiute; "Pasigo," Shoshone; "Wakamo," Warm Springs.,; "Gamooa," Wasco, Ore.; "Quamash," Umatilla, Ore.; "Camas," Nez Perce, Idaho; "Miss iss sah," Blackfeet.

Camas is the queen of all bulbs in the Inter-Mountain region. It is a member of the lily family, with a bright blue or white stalk of flowers, and a bulb covered with black bark. In Springtime when Camas is in bloom in wet meadows, the flowers grow so thickly that they look like a blue lake. After the seed is ripe, the bulbs may be dug. Old women and grandchildren usually do the digging with crooked-nosed sticks which have been hardened in fire. Bags of skin, either a small calf or deer skin hold the bulbs.

A camas feast is a community festival. For several days the sacks of bulbs have been brought in. The men's part is to bring in hard wood and green branches to roast the camas. After a day's burning of wood down to coals, the bulbs have been washed, and the coals are raked out, leaving a bed of warm ashes. This is usually about 20 feet in diameter. Green branches of alder or birch are laid down, and along the branches are placed the camas bulbs. Next a layer of ashes, then some slow coals, more ashes, more branches more camas, and so on until all the bulbs have been placed. Branches and layers of dry grass cover the top.

The camas pit is divided among four women who see to it that a supply of coals and ashes is on hand to keep the cooking going. From 24 to 36 hours is needed to complete the job. During this time, neighbors visit, sometimes deer or antelope are barbecued, and bubbling pots send forth appetizing odors.

When the camas is ready to eat, large, flat openwork willow baskets are brought to the side of the pit, and with forked sticks used as tongs, the bulbs are laid on the baskets to cool, as they are too hot to handle. When they are merely warm, the black bark is stripped from them, and the bulbs are pressed between women's hands, until they look like macaroons or ginger snaps. The fragrance is delightful like vanilla cake.

A few are eaten as dessert, but the bulk are placed in flour sacks and hung up to dry where children cannot get at them. On days when company comes, the camas is brought out as a great treat.

The taste is about like brown or maple sugar. After a few warm bulbs have been eaten, the taste cloys, but if a pickle or a piece of salt meat is eaten, the appetite returns.

There was once a war over possession of these popular bulbs. It was called the Camas War. In Idaho there is a County called Camas County, and in Montana there is Camas Prairie. In Oregon, the same bulb is called "Wakamo," and in northern California the name was "Ketten." A high valley there noted for abundance of these bulbs is still called Kettenchaw Valley.

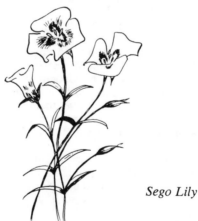

Sego Lily

SEGO LILY, Botanical name: *Calochortus Nuttalli.* Indian names: "Kok-se," Washoe; "Noona," Oregon; "Kogi," Paiute; "Segaw," Shoshone.

The Sego Lily is the State flower of Utah, because the Ute Indians taught the pioneers how to find and to eat the bulbs in starving time.

Fort Hall, Idaho has the taller Great Plains lily, which is Macrocarpus, and in the Toponz area at elev. of 8000 ft. is an unidentified lily of great beauty, which may be the Cascade Mariposa lily.

Uses: In California bulbs were formerly dug after seed had fallen and saved for winter use. In northern Nevada they were dug early in Spring, soon after the bulb thrust up its first green leaves.

The word Mariposa comes from the Spanish for the spot like the one on the petals like the spot on a butterfly's wing.

While they may seem small for digging, they grow in beds, and one can do blind digging on them after locating even one seed stalk.

VALERIAN; TOBACCO-ROOT. Botanical name: *Valeriana edulis.* Indian names: "Gwee-ya," Nevada Paiute; "Ku-ya," Northern Paiute.

This plant varies in its root, some have a root like a carrot. This is the one common to Reese River, Nevada. It is boiled, and it smells bad, but tastes good. Some people think it smells and tastes like Star Plug, hence the name, Tobacco-root.

Range use: At high elevations in rich, moist sites these plants are very leafy, and are rated high in palatability for sheep and game animals, and fair for cattle.

NUT GRASS is a cereal made from a sedge. Botanical name: *Cyperus rotundus.* Indian name: "Taboose," Paiute.

This grows in gardens that are irrigated, or where there is some natural moisture. On the rootlets of the sedge are small black tubers, size of dried currants. These are called "Taboose," and are hard and crisp when eaten raw. It tastes between fresh cocoanut and raisins. When reduced to meal and cooked as cereal, it is both nourishing and appetizing.

SAND FOOD, SAND POTATO. Botanical name: *Ammobroma sonorae.* Indian name: "Unh," Shoshone.

This is a fungus growth, a root parasite on Coldenia in desert. Eaten raw or roasted in Smoky Valley, Nevada.

WILD CARAWAY, QUEEN ANNE'S LACE, SQUAW-ROOT, TRAIL POTATO. Botanical name: *Carum Gairdneri.* Indian names: "Yampa," "Yomba," Idaho and Nevada; "Ipo," "Apaws," Oregon, also "Eppaws."

This is a wild carrot. It frequently has two finger-like roots which have a mild, nutty flavor, eaten raw. At rodeos and other Indian meetings, these Squaw-roots are sold by the tin cup full and eaten as popcorn would be.

Nevada Indians dig the roots, save them for winter, and either plain boil them or grind them into flour for puddings. Sacajawea introduced Lewis and Clark to this interesting food which was boiled and eaten as potatoes would be with meat.

Reese River Shoshones chose for the name of their newly established reservation, Yomba Reservation, in honor of this plant still so plentiful and so useful to them. This was in southern Nevada. This plant seldom occurs on the range, but in suitable spots such as moist mountain meadows, it becomes abundant.

It is found in all western states, south to California, and east to South Dakota, from a little above sea-level along the Columbia River to 9000 ft. A town in Idaho is called Yampa. Also one, in Colorado.

FAMINE FOODS

ANT PUDDING. At Owyhee, Nevada, Western Shoshone Reservation. In times when food was scarce, Indian women went out where the ants had large ant-hills to gather them before the ants were awake. They would be found clinging to sticks in clumps. A floursack was taken along to contain the ants so they could be readily seen. They were scraped off into the sack, and after looking them over for bits of earth, they are tossed in an old basket with slow coals. This heat dries the legs and pincers, so they will fall off when sifted.

Then the clean ants are browned in a skillet with flour and hot water added to make gravy. As the informant said: "Early days Indians had no starvation needs, because we used everything."

There were many foods not used in times of plenty, which were held in reserve in bad years, among them being seeds Giant Rye, (*Elymus condensatus*), wire grass, "Sineva," and the poor sunflower, in Nevada.

In northern California, a black moss, (*Alectoria Fremontii*) called "Wa-kamwa" in Oregon, no known California name. It was dried, ground and made into soup. It usually grew on conifers, but was said to taste like acorns.

Inner bark of cottonwoods and aspens was used for man and horses in hard times. Some Indians preferred it because of its sweetness.

At Elko, Nevada, in early days the Old People burned off thorns of Opuntias, cactus, and roasted pieces and stems for food. "Wogaybe."

HONEY PLANTS. Hundreds of plants give nectar for honey, especially Bee plants, wild buckwheats, and sagebrush of all kinds. The great green gentian, (*Frasera speciosa*), Elk lily of the Arapahos, is a valued plant for honey in the high mountains.

About the only flower harmful to bees is the buckeye, and if bees visit the buckeye and carry it home to the hive, it will kill the young brood.

BEVERAGES

RUSSET BUFFALO BERRIES. Thornless (*Lepargyrea canadensis*). These make a pleasant foaming drink called "Soopalallie" by Northwest Indians.

INDIAN TEA, MORMON TEA, JOINT FIR (*Ephedra spp.*). In Nevada the slender twigs are dried and an aromatic tea is used as a beverage. Paiutes call this "Tsurupe." Shoshones parch and coarsely grind ripe seeds for Indian coffee.

WHITE SAGE (*Eurotia lanata*), "Sissop." Leaves used as general beverage and to wash hair.

THREE-LOBED SUMAC (*Rhus trilobata*), Lemonade and sugar bush. The bright red berries are used for a drink.

WILD ROSE (*Rosa spp*), "Pat sur malle," Washoe. Tea from the roots makes a pretty rose colored drink.

YERBA BUENA (*Micromeria chamissonis*). Leaves dried for aromatic tea. This is the plant the original name of San Francisco came from.

It is commonly believed that Indians nowadays are eating as white people do, and while this is true of those who live near towns or on Reservations, particularly near the Rocky Mountains there are many tribes whose older members prefer their old-time foods, and who pass many happy hours in the open, collecting and preparing plants and fruits in the Indian way.

I spent years in U.S. Indian Service, studying range plants in their relation to Indian cattle and sheep projects.

Frequently these same range plants were of wide use to the Indians who were the first conservationists.

Conservation means "use, not abuse." The wise use of plants on reservations was common with Indians. Many Indians would not collect seeds and bulbs of a food plant at the same place, for fear of destroying the food supply.

When Indians killed a game animal: buffalo, deer, elk or mountain goat, every part of it was used. The hair was saved to stuff pack-saddle bags, or to put under robes for beds, the brains went to tan hides, hides went to make tepees, parfleches, which are rawhide boxes in which to carry meat, dried berries or robes—hoofs and horns were boiled down for glue, the long threads of sinew which come out of the tenderloin were saved for sewing on of beads, and even the liquid of the eyes was used to mix mineral paint to proper thickness.

Had it been left to the Indian, the buffalo would not have been destroyed.

Cultivation of fields and prairies has resulted in the destruction of many native foods.

FEASTS

After considering all the items which go to make up Indians' diet it is time to think of the feasts which make up so joyous a part of Indian life.

The regular feasts which took place yearly were spread over three seasons: Spring, Fall and Winter. Summer was too busy a time, collecting material for a Fall re-union.

One of the most interesting Spring festivals in northern California was the Acorn Feast. This was held on the first full moon after acorns were in bloom. It was a prayer for a good crop of acorns, and there was dancing and singing in the feathered costumes, common to that area. It was a natural excuse for a gathering of friends, who came bringing contributions of salmon, venison and dried berries for puddings.

Time was no object to these happy people. The first day was a rehearsal of dances, and waiting for others who came from a great distance. The second day was the Big Day, with all the trimmings of a great feast, while the third day was a review for late-comers who welcomed a chance to share the acorn soup, so symbolic of their way of life. Using everything that Nature gave them, wasting nothing, sharing all, and giving thanks.

Camas Feasts of Shoshones and Nez Perces, and Root Feasts of Warm Springs, Oregon, Indians have been described. Huckleberry Feasts of these same people were held in early Fall, when huckleberries ripened.

In Nevada and throughout the Inter-Mountain region, when a girl becomes of marriageable age, her parents gave a feast for her, much like the coming-out party of white people. This feast naturally was followed later by a wedding feast.

In Utah, the Bear Dance was a very interesting ceremony. An enclosure was made of branches around a hard-packed dance ground. In the background were camps of the families whose young folks came to dance. The dance took place at night. The dancers formed in two lines, as for Virginia reel, men and women, hand in hand. Dancing was forward and back, to the accompaniment of music made by four or five older men who alternately beat on logs with rods, or sawed with notched sticks on an old washtub, while they continually sang the same refrain.

Young men or girls who took part in the dance were indicating that they would accept a suitable offer of marriage. Sometimes couples disappeared. It was then understood that they were interested in each other. If they did not marry, no reproach was heard. There would be another Bear Dance, next Spring.

The dance floor was dimly lighted by the moon, or by the flickering smoky flames of the sitting fires of pinyon or juniper knots in front of the camps. Sometimes a mischievous boy would turn on car lights, from one of the few automobiles, but this was frowned upon as being wasteful.

A special kind of moccasin was worn by the girls. These were of white buckskin, almost to the knee, and brightly beaded. A girl who showed anxiety to be married at another time, could have it said of her: "She has on her Bear-Dance moccasins."

The term Bear Dance is said to come from the imitation of a clumsy dancing bear, courting. The Feast for this dance was in charge of the Bear Dance Boss who took charge of all contributions, from store-bought cookies and pop, to meat of any kind, except bear meat, which is seldom eaten by Indians, who think that the bear was once a man, who for his sins, was changed into a bear.

During World War Two, when Indian servicemen were home on furlough, Victory dances were held for the safety and victory of our arms, and there were the natural feasts and celebrations at those times. On Warm Springs Reservation, Oregon, a Give-away was part of these occasions. Any one desiring to honor these heroes, could bring gifts, which were put on a pile. Only the young man's name was attached to each gift. It was considered unnecessary to put on the giver's name. It looked like bragging.

Feasts were given to close family friends to celebrate recovery from a long illness. On these occasions, the house was emptied, medicinal herbs burned for fumigation, and sometimes as was seen in southern Arizona, the Medicine Man and his corps of assistants, properly painted, sang and danced inside and outside the house, eventually making gestures of "throwing the sickness away." The convalescent person was carried out into the sunshine before these rites began. The feast necessarily was confined to easily digested foods and delicacies.

In the old, old Buffalo days one man was appointed to serve as Captain of the hunt. Part of his duty was to distribute the meat equally, so that widows and old people who had no one to hunt for them got as much as they needed. Thus was carried out the Indian's motto: "One eat—all eat."

Perhaps more than any other race, the Indian has kept his sense of being one of a group. An action which affects one Indian in a way, affects all of his tribe or his clan. Generosity is part of their regular life. Any meal that is shared with friends becomes a feast with Indians.

On the west coast of the United States there are runs of salmon, surf fish and mackerel. These runs are greatly valued by the Oregon Indians. At the falls of the Columbia at Celilo the Indians have a treaty with the U.S. Government, that they can always fish there unmolested, and no one can fish there but Indians.

Just now there is legislation pending regarding the building of dam which would put an end to this fishing, with some compensation to the Indians, but that is for the future.

(NOTE: This has now been done. Indians have received compensation and Celilo is no more.)

At present there is an Indian village on the riverbank, and during the salmon run the sheds that open towards the great river are thick with drying fish which hang in pink rows above slow fires which make smoke to keep flies away.

After the fish heads are cut off, and the entire skin is pulled off like a glove, the old women with very sharp knives take out a strip along the back-bone. Peeled sharp sticks of osier dogwood are put in each fish at the top to keep the two sides from swinging in together. Any bits of fish that are broken off are carefully saved for "sugar salmon"; these bits are slightly smoked till dry and then pounded coarsely with dried berries and saved for old people to eat, or for a special company dish.

On either bank of Celilo Falls are great cliffs against which spray beats ceaselessly. Indian fishermen poise themselves upon these rocks, with long poles attached to dip nets. These nets are usually made on a barrel hoop. As the salmon jump the Falls, the Indians cast the net so as to catch the fish if he fails to go up. Sometimes two fish are caught in the same cast. Some Indians strip to a breechclout, for this work, and nearly all go barefoot as shoes slip on the wet rocks. Some of the old fellows put ropes around their waists, and tie to a rocky spur, but the young ones never bother.

Surf fish, smelt or eulachon, run up the West Coast of United States in schools. They are small and silvery. At times they are so numerous, close to shore, that Indian women wade out and scoop them up in their wide petticoats. Sometimes the fish are so fat when hung up and smoked that they drip grease, then they are called candlefish.

In northern California, the river which drains the most country is called Eel River, because of the quantities of eels which run up that stream. These are not ordinary eels. They have holes along the first six inches of their bodies, beginning at the head. They are called Lamprey eels, and in ancient Rome lampreys were considered a great delicacy.

A regular Spring festival among Hoopa and Klamath Indians is an eel roast usually held on the river-bank. Sometimes a basket trap is set in the river. The open-work basket has a funnel of basket work inside the big basket. The basket is so anchored in the stream that the eels will push their way into the funnel, as they swim up-stream. Their weight opens the sides and releases them into the big basket from which they cannot escape.

This eel roast took place after the first high water which brought up salmon. There were rites for First Salmon in both California and Oregon.

FISHING WITHOUT HOOKS OR SPEARS

Sometimes when Indians were traveling, fish were seen in pools, certain plants were mashed up raw and put into these pools. The fish would float to the surface and could be skimmed out with sieves of willow. Blue curls (*Trichostema lanceolatum*); turkey mullein (*eremocarpus setigerus*); soap root (*chlorogallum pomeridianum*), and sometimes fresh leaves or nuts of buckeye. This said to be poisonous, but if the fish are put into fresh water, they recover, unharmed. Some authorities think the stellate hairs on Blue curls and turkey mullein, get into the fish's gills and hold them open, so in time he would drown. The writer has seen these two used successfully by Indians.

Throughout the reservations just west of the Rocky Mountains there are many berries and other fruits which are much relished by Indians.

Fruits eaten raw or cooked of the following: Buckberry, or Wolfberry, Lycium species, with bright red acid berries, used in puddings, first cooked and seeds strained out through a willow sieve.

BUFFALO or BULL BERRY, botanical name: *Elaegnus argentea*. The silver buffalo berry grows in thickets. Makes a handsome hedge, as the thorny branches interlace, and stand pruning well. Berries are bright red, but the bush is pure silver. Berries are eaten raw, made into jelly or dried.

Indian names: Arapaho: "Auch ha hay be na" refers to the Russet Buffalo berry, thornless, with brown, ripe berries. Oregon Indian name for this one is "Soopolallie." Makes a foaming drink. Botanical name: *Lepargyrea canadensis*.

The Indian names of Silver Buffalo berry are: "Wea pu wi," Yerington, Nevada, Paiute; "Weyumb," Smoky Valley and Elko Shoshone; "Me e Nixen," Blackfeet.

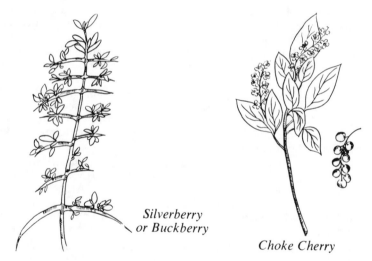

Silverberry
or Buckberry

Choke Cherry

CHOKECHERRIES: Botanical names: *Prunus demissa,* also *P. melanocarpa.* Indian names: "Daw esha bui," refers to jelly, "Dongeszip," whole bush; both of these Shoshone and Paiute. "Tamash," bush, Warm Springs, "T'mish" cherries, same "Tsam-chit," Washoe.

Uses: Indians eagerly seek the fruit throughout the Intermountain region, and inland on Coast States for use, fresh, dried and in jelly or syrup. Dried cherries are also used with elk, deer meat and back fat in making of pemmican.

Chokecherry biscuits are made from dried chokecherries, from which bits of stone have been removed, dried on flat baskets. Turned daily till dry, given to babies for stomach ache.

Wild currants are most abundant and beautiful near Owyhee, Nevada. There are red ones, golden ones, and black ones, used chiefly for jelly and for drying.

GOLDEN CURRANT. Botanical name: *Ribes aureum*. Indian name: "Bogumbe," Shoshone; "Pokops,' Paiute; "Mobabuwi," Yerington Paiutes.

BLACK CURRANT. Botanical name: *Ribes petiolare*. Indian name: "Owa pawump," Shoshone; "Non hal wa," Washoe.

WAX CURRANT, BEAR CURRANT. Botanical name: *Ribes cereum*. Indian names: "Tsapuwi," Paiute; "Skee yap," Warm Springs, Ore.; "Wood un de kan," Shoshone; "Dembogem," Shoshone, Tonopah.

Wax or Bear currants grow right beside the golden currants. They have a sticky dry taste, not much juice. Too many are emetic. Indians say that the reason they are called Bear currants, is because the bear who likes berries saw people eating all his favorite fruits, and he put this taste in Bear Currants so people would not want to eat them.

ELDERBERRY. Botanical name: *Sambucus glauca*. Indian name: "Hubu," Paiute; Warm Springs, Ore., "Muth'p," the berries. This is the blue elderberry. Ripe fruits used. Medicinal uses too.

ELDERBERRY. Botanical name: *Sambucus racemosa*. Indian name: "Koono gibu," Paiute; "Duhiembuh," Shoshone. This is the red elderberry, not very palatable. Medicinal uses.

BLACK HAWTHORN, HAW BUSH. Botanical name: *Crataegus Columbiana*. Indian names: "Simnasho," Warm Springs, Ore.; "We nap ish," Bannock.

There is an Indian village called Simnasho in Oregon, this is a corruption of "Ashnum asho," the Warm Springs name for this hawthorn. These Indians gathered the fruit after it had dried and been frosted on the bushes, and used it as others use the Sarvis Berry. It is quite seedy. Great thickets of Simnasho border the stream in that little valley.

ROSE SPECIES. Especially *Rosa Nutkana,* also *Rosa Spaldingii,* named for Idaho's early missionary, who first reported it near Lapwai. "Tsiavi," Shoshone and Paiute; "Pat sur malle," Washoe; "Yano," Arapaho.

Uses: Northern Indians such as Blackfeet and Rocky Boy children use the fruit which is very large and very fragrant to eat raw or to make jelly of. Washoes eat berries raw.

"Ska pash-wee" is Warm Springs name for bush. It means "Mean old lady she sticks you."

SERVICE BERRY, SARVIS BERRY, SHAD-BLOW, botanical name: *Amelanchier alnifolia*. Indian name: "Tuambe," (Note: "Tuambe" name given the writer by Fort Hall Indians.) "Tuyembee," Shoshone. "Saskatoon," British Columbia; "Ok a nook," Blackfeet.

Purplish black fruit used both fresh and dried by Indians and early settlers, for eating and for pemmican.

Cactus fruits of many varieties are gathered when ripe.

PRICKLY PEAR. Botanical name: *Opuntia Engelmanni*. Indian name: "Navoo," Shoshone.

LADY FINGER. Botanical name: *Mammillaria*. Indian name "Tso-ha," Shoshone.

PEYOTE. Indian name: "Wogaybe," Shoshone. This is not eaten as fruit would be, but a tea is made from dried sections, and is drunk to induce visions.

GREENS

After a long hard winter with highly starchy foods or meat, Indians welcomed the coming of Spring, and the appearance of green shoots of cow-parsnip (Indian Rhubarb), ferns, wild celery and the first leaves of sunflower. These were carefully cooked about as asparagus would be.

Added to the foregoing should be the stalks of Indian Balsam (*Leptotaenia multifida*), Indian name "Toza."

On Warm Springs Reservation, Oregon, stalks of wild celery are still peeled and eaten fresh, while the seeds are used for seasoning soups, etc. For miles there, these are the only plants growing in heavy red adobe soil. The plants are called: "P-tish, p-tish," while the stalk below the umbel is called "Cumsee."

In the same area, the stalks of wild sunflower are eaten while they snap readily, while the roots are barbecued.

INDIAN LETTUCE, MINER'S LETTUCE, botanical name: *Claytonia perfoliata*. Succulent leaves, perforated by the stem, growing under oaks, may be eaten raw or cooked with lambs quarter or mustard for greens in California.

In desert country, notably in Nevada, Golden Prince's Plume, Indian cabbage, botanical name: *Stanleya pinnata,* is quite abundant, and is visible for long distances on account of its beautiful plumy blossoms. This plant has a large bunch of basal leaves of cabbage texture. It is useful when cooked, but several waters must be poured off, before it is safe to eat. It is highly emetic otherwise.

CLOVER in northern California was formerly eagerly eaten by Indians. Particularly liked was *Trifolium virescens,* called Bear clover by some. Its tendency to bloat is offset by dipping leaves or flowers into salt water.

CAT-TAIL, botanical name: *Typha latifolia*. Indian name: "Tabu'oo," Paiute; "Toiba," Washoe.

The end of a new stem of cat-tail is popular with Washoes.

PEANUT-BUTTER PLANT. Botanical name: *Glyptopleura marginata*. Indian name: "Cumi-segee," Paiute. Another common name is Rabbitguts because the under side of plant looks like an opened rabbit. Leaves eaten raw, are deliciously like peanut butter greens. Pyramid Lake, Nevada.

MEAT

Meat has always been the most highly valued food that an Indian could have. Some tribes, such as the Blackfeet in Montana, depended almost entirely on meat for food. The buffalo furnished them besides meat, hides for tepees, and for clothing and robes, hair for pillows and for saddle stuffing, sinews for sewing. Bladders and intestines were used for containers.

Horns of buffalo were highly polished for ornaments in head-dresses, and elk horns were carved into spoons with delicately shaped handles.

After game animals were cut up into quarters, odd bits of meat were cut into strips and jerked by drying in the open air. This was called jerked meat or "jerky." Some jerky is cut with the grain and some across the grain. Some Indians make a salt brine with pepper in it, and the strips are quickly dipped into this, and then hung on racks above a fire, made with green or damp wood to make a slow smoke. This to keep flies and yellow-jackets away.

Plains Indians took the dry hide of a mule-deer and opened it out to make an Indian suit-case. When it was filled with dried meat, berries dried, or personal belongings, the deer legs and both end were folded over, just as the flaps of an envelope are folded to make a rawhide box, flat and easy to carry on horseback. Rawhide lacings keep the box shut. These boxes are called parfleches, and were originally intended to carry extra arrows. Fleche is the French word for arrows. In Hudson Bay Company employ were many Canadians. In the far North many Indian families have French names, because of Frenchmen who married Indian women.

PEMMICAN, called "Makakin" in Blackfeet and "Wasna" in Sioux was the invention of the Indians. It is a mixture of finely ground meat, back fat, (*depouiller*), and dried berries. It used to be packed solidly in skin bags made of calf hide, or a stomach lining.

A hundred pound sack of pemmican had so much nourishment in it that it would feed four men for thirty days, with no other food. It would be much used by trappers and Mountain men during the time when Hudson Bay Company ruled the North country, while travel was as yet entirely by horse or pack train.

NUTS

In California acorns figured very largely in Indians' diet. There are many kinds of oak trees, and acorns varied in size and shape.

Black oak acorns were the favorites in northern California. Tan oak acorns came next, and white oaks last. When acorns were gathered each kind was kept separate, but preparation was the same for all. The acorns were soaked over night, which caused the shell to split open. Old women then picked out the kernels. Even the blind ones could do this. The nuts were spread on open work baskets to dry and when they were dry enough, they were ground to flour in a stone mortar.

If acorn soup was desired, it was made about like thin gruel. A few tribes made acorn bread. It was made up in round loaves, and before it was baked, it was a pale brick-red color. If baked in ashes, the bread was wrapped in fern leaves, when the slow heat turned the bread black and with the fern prints on it, looked like a piece of coal with marks of fossils.

Some tribes added red clay to the acorn meal when making acorn bread in proportion of 1 to 20, to make a stiff dough. Chemists state that the iron in the red clay helps offset the over-amount of protein in the acorns. Bread is remarkably sweet.

After the acorn meal was ground, it was leached to take the bitterness out in the following manner: a frame was prepared with incense cedar twigs laid overlapping, like shingles on a roof, the acorn meal was spread out on the frame, and water poured through the meal repeatedly, until the meal turned pink, when it was dried and kept until used. The cedar twigs gave a spicy taste to the meal.

Long ago, a sort of Indian penicillin was made by covering the acorn meal closely, to make it sweat and mold. When the skin of the mold was firm enough to roll up, it was peeled off and kept in a damp place. If anyone had a boil or bad sore, this mold was applied to draw out the inflammation.

Pinyons or Pine Nuts are common in parts of California, Utah, Nevada, Arizona and New Mexico. The nuts are small and soft-shelled. Nuts of the Digger Pine are hard shelled and larger than the pinyons. These nuts mean much to the Indians who gather them for sale, and they form a large part of Indian diet. Especially is pine nut harvest a season of great rejoicing. Families camp out for weeks at a time, gathering not only pine-nuts but various plant medicines which ripen at the same time. The pinyon cones are usually roasted before the nuts are eaten, and nut surplus is buried until needed.

The life of many a motherless Indian baby has been saved by feeding it pine-nut soup, used as milk would be.

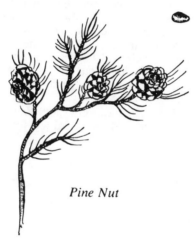

Pine Nut

In northern California, hazel nuts are highly valued, not only for the nuts which taste much like filberts, but the bush that bears them has wood that can be split very fine, and it is used in the finest basketry.

In the same area, the nuts of California Bay, called pepperwood nuts, contain a great deal of oil, and have a spicy taste. They are roasted and used as condiments, also eaten with clover in the Spring, to avert bloat.

BUCKEYES (*Aesculus Californica*). These nuts which belong to the horse-chestnut family are poisonous until roasted. Following the roasting, the nuts are reduced to meal, which is placed in a clear pool of running water for days. The pool has a bottom of sand. Water runs in and out. Each day a stick is laid on the bank. After ten days the meal is taken out and cooked, or in some places, hot stones are put in the pool to cook it. As this spoils soon, it is eaten at once.

SWEET COLTSFOOT, YUKI SALT PLANT. Botanical name: *Petasites palmata*. In early days, before the white man came, Indians who lived far from the ocean, needed salt.

There is a plant in northern California, a salt plant. Its botanical name palmata comes from the large leaves, size of a man's hand, with outspread fingers. The plant has long stems. It grows in shady places in the redwood belt.

Indians gathered the big leaves and stems in quantity, and brought them home, and spread them out in the hot sun to wilt. When the leaves were limber, each one was rolled into a tight ball. The stems were treated in the same manner. Then the balls were placed on a thick piece of redwood bark, with slow coals around it, and placed where the wind could not scatter it. With this slow heat, the leafballs were changed into ashes which were almost pure salt. This salt was used with soup or anything but meat.

SEEDS

Among cereals made from plant seeds, that made from Balsam root Sunflower seeds (*Balsamorrhiza sagittata*) is very tasty. Ripe seeds are spread on the ground, fire is dropped among them, and stirred around with a stick. The fire will go out and only the seeds will be left. These are put in a willow basket-sieve, and charcoal is sifted out. Then the seeds are put in a flat basket, and are shaken and blown, and everything but the seeds is carried away. Then the seeds are ground. The meal is stirred into boiling water, and made into mush. This will have a toasted or popcorn flavor.

Indian names: "Ah'Kerh," Shoshone; "Sugilatse," Washoe; "Po'Ah, Kerh," the green leaved one; "Kosiak," the gray one, Shoshone; "Pe-ak" or "Pe-ik," Northern Paiute.

WHITE SUNFLOWER, "Pe-ak," Owyhee Paiutes, make a pudding from the ground seed meal, and add sweet fruited juniper berries for a gala dish.

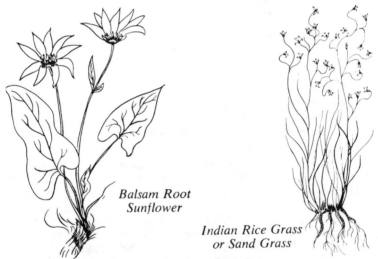

*Balsam Root
Sunflower*

*Indian Rice Grass
or Sand Grass*

SAND GRASS, INDIAN RICE GRASS, botanical name, *Oryzopsis hymenoides*. Indian names: "Wye," Paiute and Shoshone. This bunchgrass is of great value in desert country, because it will grow without water in pure sand. It is very important to Indian life, because it furnishes food for man and beast. The seed, which is black and round, is gathered by hand by the women of the tribe. Bunches are caught in one hand and a sharp sickle cuts the bunches, which are then tossed on a canvas. If the seed is to be used in re-planting the range, bunches are beaten with wooden flails. If seed is to be used for food, a match is touched to the light stems, and they burn up leaving clean seed. Burning might destroy the life in the seed which is to be planted.

Paiute Indians have large shallow baskets, shaped like clamshells. These are called winnowers. The seeds are poured onto the baskets, which are shaken sidewise. A tap of the finger on the bottom makes bits of earth, straw or unripe seeds seek the edge of the basket where they are easily pushed over. Sometimes, when the seeds are nearly cleaned, the contents are poured onto a canvas from a standing position, and any light chaff is gone with the wind, thus leaving remaining seed absolutely clean.

This seed is ground as needed into meal for mush. It is light gray, the meal—in color, and is about the thickness of Cream of Wheat. It has high food value.

In re-seeding Sand Grass in the desert where it has been killed out by over-grazing, the seed is broadcast among the sagebrush in strips about four feet wide, with a four foot strip left between sowings that the wind may carry seed and fill in the space. In order to keep birds from picking up the seed, sheep may be driven over it. Their little hoofs cover it with soil as they scuff along.

A tribal enterprise, conducted by the Paiute women of Walker River Reservation, Nevada, was the collecting of Sand Grass seed in 1936, for re-seeding on other reservations. It did well at Pyramid Lake, Nevada, and on Fort Hall Reservation, Idaho, where it was native, but had been killed out by over grazing.

INDIAN GRAVY: A tiny Blazing Star (*Mentzelia albicaulis*), is known to Paiutes as the Gravy plant. This seed is red. It is put into a hot frying pan, and when seed turns darker red, warm water is added and it is stirred till it thickens. This plant is called "Ku-Ha." Seed of the large Evening Star, *Mentzelia laevicaulis* is similarly used.

SCREW BEAN, a form of mesquite, botanical name: *Prosopis pubescens.* Indian name: "Quier," Moapa Paiute, beans pounded for food.

HONEY MESQUITE, botanical name: *Prosopis juliflora*, "Ah Pee," Moapa, similarly used.

PINOLE: This is the name given to meal made from small grass seeds or weed seeds, or wild flower seeds. Buttercup seeds, lambs' quarter or goosefoot seeds were also used. These were first put through a basket sieve, and later cleaned with a winnower by standing at the house corner, or any other windy point, and pouring into another basket. The clean seeds were then placed in an old stout closely woven basket with slow coals and tossed. Heat cause the seed husks to fly off, and the semi-roasting gave the seeds a popcorn flavor.

Seeds were then ground in a stone mortar, and sifted. A small cup sized closely woven basket held the meal, now called Pinole. This was passed around to guests, and pinches were taken with the fingers. This was regarded as a delicacy, and was never cooked, nor eaten with salt.

Not far north of Ukiah, California, is a small Indian village called Pinoleville, in recognition of this favorite food of the Pomo Indians.

In Nevada, several members of the Mustard family furnish orange colored seeds, which are carefully collected and ground to make gravy, by adding hot water to the meal. One variety of wild mustard seldom sets seed. The Indian name given to this one means: "Old Maid Sister."

For seed collection most tribes use a cornucopia-shaped basket tightly woven. This is held in the left hand, close to the ground, while the right hand uses a seed-beater, made of willow, and shaped like a pancake turner, to strike the plant and beat the seeds into the basket.

Among Nevada Indians, it was possible to learn about plants from the seeds if the plant's leaves were gone, but seed-pods remained. My name among these Indians was "Bahai wakidu," the Seed-Seeker.

CHIA. This is a sage. Botanical name: *Salvia Columbariae*. Seeds roasted, ground into meal, water added to make gruel. In early days in northern California, runners carried ripe seeds in belt pouches and ate them en route. Pomo Indians ground seeds for pinole. Chia is the Spanish name for this plant. Cortez found Mexican natives using these seeds parched and ground into meal. Jepson states that Mission fathers used an infusion of seeds for fevers and for cooling drinks. The '49ers used the seeds for gun-shot wounds, in a poultice.

CORN. Following is a quotation from "The Arickaras" ed. by John C. Ewers, "From 1804 on, some cultivation was done by Indians on small patches of corn on the Missouri bottom . . . work done altogether by women, and entirely by hoes, corn, pumpkins and squashes."

"This corn is said to be the original kind discovered in America. The stalk seldom exceeds 2½ or 3 ft. in height, and the ears form a cluster near the surface of the ground . . . Grain is small, hard, and covered with a thicker shell than that raised in warmer climates. Yield about 20 bushels to the acre. When green . . . it is slightly boiled after which it is dried, shelled and laid by . . . will keep any length of time."

Preparing corn, drying, as still done on Montana and Wyoming reservations: Take corn while it still has milk when pricked. Take two ears and tie them together by husks. Have a wash-boiler with water at a full rolling boil, with a broomstick laid across. Put in the corn across the stick, and boil 8 minutes. Take it out and hang on a clothes-line, several days, covering at night. Hang up in a store-room when completely dry. When wanted for dinner, cook till warmed through. Even the cobs retain sweetness.

Corn is the most important food plant domesticated by the Indian.

Method used by Papago Indians, Arizona: Shell dry corn. Have a fire of mesquite wood burned down to coals. Have some large, old baskets. Put in some slow coals or very hot ashes. Put in the corn and toss it, so it does not burn. It will have an odor like popcorn, and the husks will fly off. When done, grind in an Indian mortar, fine as corn meal, and it can be cooked as cereal.

Governor Bradford referring to Squanto, an Indian chief, told how he came to the relief of the Pilgrim Fathers, with corn, showing them how to plant it, and to put a fish head in each hill, to fertilize the ground. Ground should be worked when leaves on the oaks were no bigger than a squirrel's ear.

CORN: Indian name: Conohana, a Cherokee Indian dish.

1 pint English walnuts (black are better), 1 short quart cooked corn, 3 pints cooked hominy. Cook the walnuts in a little water and hominy juice until they are soft enough to be crushed with a fork. Then add the cooked corn and cooked hominy, and a piece of butter, size of a walnut. Salt to taste. Stew until seasoned, put in a pan and bake brown.

Seeds of plants used for seasoning only:

WILD CELERY: Botanical name: *Apium species*. Indian names: "Hobe," Shoshone; "Yeduts," Paiute; "Mo-zook-addas," Washoe.

SWEET ANISE: Botanical name: *Osmorrhiza occidentalis*. Indian name: "Bossowey," Paiute and Shoshone.

GROUND PLUMS: Botanical name: *Astragalus species*. Indian name: "Namadagide," Paiute.

PEPPERMINT; PENNYROYAL; SPEARMINT; SWEET SAGE (*Artemisia dracunculoides*), "Pawots," Shoshone. Seeds of all above steeped and added to dishes for flavoring.

POND LILY (*Nuphar polysepalum*). On Klamath Marsh are about 10,000 acres of this great golden water lily. It was formerly harvested by the women with dugouts poling slowly along, and pulling the pods off their stems. The days harvest was brought to shore and emptied into a hole where fermentation ensued for weeks or until the end of the season, when the heap was stirred up and the best seeds brought up and dried and subsequently roasted. When ground these seeds make a fine cereal, but the preparation is difficult. "Wokas," Klamath name.

Throughout northern California there are many little mountain lakes far removed from the great Klamath country, but every one has its share of yellow lilies, not now used as food.

TARWEED. There are several varieties of this plant, called tarweeds because of their intense stickiness. They seed abundantly, and are agreeably aromatic and oily, form an important part of the small seeds used for pinole in northern California.

THE SALT JOURNEY

NOTE by the author: This account has been previously given in an article entitled: "Out of the Past" by Lucy Young and myself, which was published by California State Historical Quarterly in December, 1941.

Lucy Young was a very old full-blood Indian of northern California, who related this story to me as we traveled horseback through the Wilderness Area of Mendocino National Forest. The story has an account of the Salt Journey made yearly by Indians to procure their year's supply of salt.

"There were certain salt springs in the neighborhood of North Yolla Bolly Mountain which were under the claimed ownership of Indians who were hostile to Lucy's tribe. Because they had no horses, Lucy's people, the entire journey was made on foot. . . . Old people, very small children and nursing mothers were left at home. If stores of roots and berries had been left over from the winter, these were buried in pits in the ground, or placed in safe caches.

Big baskets or surplus valuables were hung securely in trees. The summer would be dry, and there were no thieves in those days. If possible, fresh meat was obtained in order to leave some with the stay-at-homes, and in order to take some with the Salt party for the first day or two, when hunting was unlikely to be good.

The journey was planned to take a month's time, reaching the Salt Country, so as to arrive close to North Yolla Bolly about full moon.

Knee-length buckskin moccasins were worn by the big walking children, i.e., those able to take care of themselves, and carry a small pack of salt as well. The woman, too, wore moccasins, but the men went barefoot.

For some time before the journey began, old baskets, nets and carriers of any kind were collected and patched so that they could contain salt. Lattice work was made to fit in the baskets to hold successive layers of salt.

As they traveled, they lived off the country, with frequent pauses to fish or hunt, to dry meat, or to prospect for bulbs, or to mark the places where they grew, with the thought of harvesting them when they were ripe, on the return trip.

Having finally arrived at the Salt Ground, they waited, if too early, for the moon to be right. Some of the women kept the children with their baskets on the edge of No-Mans-Land—the section between the territory claimed for hunting by Chief Lassik, Lucy's great -uncle and the Salt Country, claimed by their enemies—while the swift runners among the women, and the entire band of warriors crept on to the Salt Country.

There, crusts of salt covered the ground, and frequently low hanging shrubs were encrusted also and could be stripped quickly into the baskets. The moon made it light as day. If the time was exactly right, they were not molested, but if they were a day or more, late, their passage was fiercely disputed by the other Indians.

If they were lucky, their foray was successful, and it resulted in nearly a year's supply of salt, which, when they had put a discreet distance between them and their enemies, they would stop to pick over for sticks and stones, and sometimes boil down in baskets with hot stones, pouring off the small dirt on top, and leaving a crust of pure salt to be skimmed off when cold.

Secure in the possession of this valuable salt, much hunting was done on the way home, meat was dried, and fish was dried and smoked. Frequently they met other hunting parties, and much visiting and sharing of game ensued.

Small wonder that all Indians thought of Heaven as "The Happy Hunting Ground!" It was an ideal life—that of the Salt Journey—making use of everything in Nature, wasting nothing, sharing everything, stealing nothing.

Why steal? When anything could be had for the asking? Compare this life with the ten years following the coming of the white man, when an Indian had no rights that a white man was bound to respect, not even the Indian's wife, or life, or land, or game.

Small wonder that reprisals and bloody battles such as Lucy Young witnessed, were common events in the years that followed.

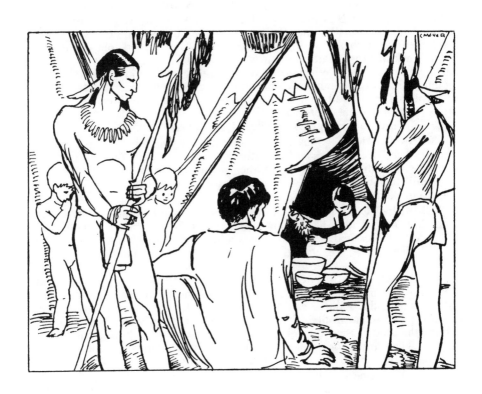

RECIPES OF INDIAN FOODS

Recipes of Indian Foods, by Myrtle Shaw (now Mrs. New Moon), Carson Indian School girl, of Stewart, Nevada.

Note: by Mrs. Murphey, these recipes were exhibited at First Annual Flower show, May 30-31, 1935, Stewart, Nevada. Used by permission of Mrs. New Moon.

Indian Recipes: These are recipes which the Nevada Paiutes still use.

WILD CHOKE CHERRIES: Known to Paiutes as "Daw-esha-boi." Ripe in summer, sometimes early Fall. They grow on mountains along streams. After picked from bushes, they are washed thoroughly in tubs of water. They are similar to grapes and plums. Can also be stored away as desserts for winter. Also cooked to make jam or preserves. When ready to cook: First, let it cook for so many hours. Smash it after cooked. Take seeds out. Make into preserves or jam. Eaten as a fruit between meals.

WILD BUCK or BUFFALO BERRIES: Pick in July and August. They are small in size, smaller than beans. Contain little seeds. Grow upon a gray leaved thorny bush, six to twelve feet tall. After picked, put out to dry for one week or more. Put into flour sacks and store away for winter. Cook to make sauce or jam. When the berries are ready to cook: First take any amount of berries and put over open fire, or either on stove. After boiled, put through sieve. Add sauce, made of flour and water. Sweeten. These berries are found along riversides or near water.

Note: This is a Lepargyrea, or Silver Buffalo berry.

SKUNK BERRIES: Pick in early summer, around June. These berries are red. Place in sun to dry. Keep stirring. Let it dry for one week. Pick over after it is dryed and wash. Either pound or grind. Boil and strain. Cook until the juice is red. Add meat grease and sweeten. Add cornmeal flavor to thicken.

TUMBLE-WEED, "Sunu." Late summer around August. Grow out on the hills of Nevada. Use willow wand to get these. Pound it with stick until seeds are loosened. Take the seeds and grind. These seeds are grayish in color. The seeds are ground and eaten, or can be made into flour for bread.

WILD MOUNTAIN GRASS, called "Wye" or "Wey," in Paiute. Out in Spring, ripe in June. Grow in bunches on the hillsides. Gathered into baskets, which the Paiutes call "Kawonoo." Piled into canvas. After get so much piled, set it on fire. Stir it with sticks, so grass won't burn too fast to burn the seeds. Seed do not burn. When the grass is burnt, only seeds are left. They are black. Take and grind to make flour and sauce.

Note: This is Sand Grass, *Oryzopsis hymenoides.*

"KUHA." Ripe in latter part of June. Use same as "Wye." Grind it. Before ground, seeds are grayish-black. After ground, it is black and greasy. When it is all ground, mix with water. Stir it. Cook over open fire outside. After cooked, sweeten. It is eaten as dessert. Note: Probably a small Mentzelia.

WILD WEED MUSTARD. These weed mustard are called "Acjha." Ripe late June. Grows out on hillsides. Use willow wand and burden basket for this too. After swept into the basket, pick small weeds and leave the seeds. The seeds are small and red. This food is strong, much stronger than the other seeds. First: Stir it over the fire in a pan. Grind it. Make it into soup. Mix with ground "wye" and ground "Sunu" to take strong taste away.

WILD CURRANT. "Baw-gaw-pesha." Ripe in summer. Grows near rivers and streams. If the bush does not get enough water for its growth, then the berries are sweet. Method of cooking: Wash the berries. Boil with water. After cooked, strain the juice, to make it into jelly. Save the berries to make preserves.

"HOO-TOO." Ripe in August. Found high up in the mountains. Gather into baskets. When ready to use, wash in water. Boiled. When cooked, make into jam, and eaten as dessert.

WILD POTATOES: "Ya-pah." Ripe in September. Found on the mountains. They shed pretty white flowers. After the flowers have fallen off, it signs that the potatoes are ripe. Then they are dug out. When these potatoes are ready to be dug out and used, first, wash the dirt off. Bake in hot ashes or boil like Irish potatoes. If wanted to store away for winter food, put them out in the sun to dry, then store away. After storing away, they are sweet. They have a yellowish color on the inside. Outside is similar to sweet potatoes after stored.

Note: This is also known as "Trail potato," but is "Yomba" to Shoshones. Botanical name: *Carum Gairdneri.*

INDIAN POTATOES. Fall of the year. Found along creeks. Size of an egg. Black on outside, orange color inside. Method of cooking: Wash off dirt. Boil potatoes with peelings for an hour. Cool. Do not blow on the potatoes, will get watery. Eaten same as Irish potatoes.

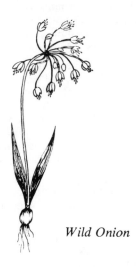

Wild Onion

LARGE WILD ONIONS, "patuse." Grow along streams. Found on mountains. Gathered in May and June. Eaten as they are found, both onions and leaves eaten. Wash in water.

INDIAN BREADS: Mix parched corn meal with meat soup and make a stiff dough. Add salt. Place bread on a 2-forked stick. Cook over hot coals.

Mix flour with baking powder and water. Have an open fire hot enough to bake the bread. Flap the dough to a middle-sized round shape. Put in hot ashes to bake. After baked, put in a clean flour sack to keep the bread from getting cold. This mixture can be baked or fried over a stove in a pan.

WILD GAME

GROUNDHOGS, "Ketu" in Paiute. They are out late summer. Found along the mountain sides. Similar to prairie dogs, only a lot bigger, the size of a tom-cat and very delicious. First, brush the dust off from the body. Then clean the inside. Have a hot fire, so when you put out the fire you'll have hot ashes to roast your meat. Put the groundhog in the hot ashes, and cover it with the ashes. Leave it to cook for half a day. After it is cooked, peel off the skin. It is then eaten as a meat dish. It is one of best and most pleasing dishes for the Paiutes.

PORCUPINE, "Cjaqutdu," is found on top and everywhere on the mountains. They can be killed any time of the year. First build a fire, then put the porcupine on fire, until the quills are burned off. Then scrape it. Dig a small hole in the ground, and build another fire in the hole. Porcupine is thrown into hot ashes and dirt. Small fire is kept burning on top. Left there overnight. Taken out in the morning and can be eaten for meals.

JACK RABBIT, "Kamu." These wild rabbits are out all seasons. Found everywhere in the sagebrushes. Best time to get these rabbits is in September. Because that is the time they are fat and are good to eat. After killed: Take the skin off. Clean the inside. Leave kidney, liver and heart. Wash the whole rabbit thoroughly. Cut in small pieces to fry, or boil to make soup. Or put over an open fire to roast. May be stored and dried for winter food.

PRAIRIE DOGS, "Kepa." These squirrels live under the ground. Usually live out in the fields and deserts. After killed: Have an open fire a-blazing. Clean the inside of the squirrels. Lay them out in a row on leaves or sagebrushes. Let the fire burn down. Put in hot ashes and cover with ashes. Keep a small fire on top. Let them cook for ten minutes. After cooked, hit with a small tree branch to take ashes off. When the squirrel is cooked, the skin is black. Before cooked the skin is gray and black. Peel the skin. These are eaten with Indian bread which is very good.

ANTELOPE, "Goipa." They live high up in rocky peaks. They're regular cliff climbers. After killed: Cut horns, head and neck off. Clean inside. Wash thoroughly. Cook on top of open fire until it browns. Either fry or it can be boiled. Eaten same as meat.

SAGE HENS (Grouse or Guinea hens). Found upon high mountains. Eaten like ducks or chickens. After killed: Take the feathers off. Clean insides. Wash thoroughly in water. Cook outside in hot ashes, or it may be fried, or boiled and made into soup.

PELICAN, "Panusa." Only the breast part is eaten. Each breast is enough to feed four people.

There is other Game which is fixed the same way as Sage hens, such as: Wild Geese, "Naguta"; Mallards, "Puhu"; Mudhens, "Soya." These three all belong to the Duck and geese family.

BIG TROUT FISH, "Agai," Big Trout Fish of Pyramid Lake, the very smallest weighing 2 lbs. and commonly 25-30 lbs, 4 ft. in length; diameter, 7-8 inches. It is lens-shaped and narrower from side to side than from back to belly. First cut the tail and head off. Clean inside. Wash. Roast in hot ashes. Add salt. After cooked, hang it outside on poles or put in a row on top of a house on canvas to dry. After dried, store away for winter. When ready to eat, no cooking to be done.

Found also at Pyramid Lake: Spring trout, "Tama-agai," 18 inches long. Black skinned fish, "Kuy-ui," 20 inches long.

Recipes for food, not plants, given by Pyramid Lake, Nevada, Children.

Child's recipe for cooking wild onions, the little ones called: "Se-e" which are reserved for little children's digging, because they are so shallowly rooted: "Se-e." Dig it. Make a fire to have hot rocks. Dig a hole, put onions in. Put hot rocks on top, earth on top of that. After two days take onion out and spread to cool, because it is still hot. Add water, stir around, and eat the onions.

BLACK-SKINNED FISH, "Quee-wee," 20 inches long, from Pyramid Lake. Take insides out where the eggs come out. Tie mouth with cloth to keep out ashes, or fill with green leaves. Roast under ashes, and when done, remove filling.

PELICAN EGGS: "Panoso-noho." First get the eggs. Boil till done.

PRAIRIE DOGS: "Gwuppa." Singe hair. Clean inside. Roast in ashes.

DEER: To cook a deer in itself. Clean the body. Cut off the legs. Take a stick and pin the neck together. Build a fire and throw some small stones into it. Cut some meat into small bits.

Next: Put water into the deer, using the ribs as a pot. Throw in the hot stones, next the small bits of meat. They will be done in four minutes. Take this small meat out, but leave rocks till they are cold, then add more hot rocks, and the meat in the pot itself will cook.

CURE FOR TB: First kill a badger. Take the fat from around the heart. Melt it. Put it in a bottle and drink it every other day.

Note: This may have a building-up effect equal to codliver oil. Also, the badger bears a great reputation for strength and courage in proportion to his size.

MEDICINAL PLANTS

Dr. Sanders, U.S.I.S. physician stationed at Carson Indian Agency, in 1937, headed his medical program, with these words:

"Poverty, Ignorance, Custom and Disease are the Four Horsemen who trample the Indian into the dust. They cannot be combated singly, for they ride four abreast, and a victory over one is a triumph over all."

Because more time was spent in Nevada than anywhere else, more information has been given on Nevada plants, also these Indians live more primitively than many others, and were willing to share their knowledge with the writer, with the thought that it would not be lost, but made a matter of record.

Three Indian tribes occupy Nevada with an Indian population of about six thousand: Washoe, Paiute and Shoshone.

Washoes occupy colonies near Gardnerville and Reno, and also spend six months of every year at their old camping ground near Lake Tahoe.

Paiutes are scattered over western and northern Nevada. They share reservations with Summit Lake and Fort MacDermitt, and have large reservations at Pyramid Lake and Walker River (Shurz).

There is also the "Burns Band" of Paiutes on the Idaho side of the State line, but included in Western Shoshone Reservation at Owyhee.

Las Vegas and Moapa Indians are classed as Southern Paiutes. Shoshones use all the rest of Nevada, with colonies near all towns, and the large reservation near the northern border extending several miles into Idaho, which is known as Western Shoshone.

Many of these Indians still depend largely upon their ancient sources of supply of native plants for medicinal, ceremonial and subsistence uses. During the course of a year, they live at several places: on the mountain, in the desert, near a school, depending upon seasons as did their ancestors, in pursuit of food, medicines, or basket material, gathering all of these as part of the women's work, while the men herd sheep, work with cattle or as hay hands in irrigated sections.

In the course of their travels they draw upon several botanical zones, whose plants vary with altitude, and from areas, which for subsistence purposes present little or nothing to the eye of a white person, but which formerly were adequate for Indians who wrested from seemingly barren surroundings something for their every need.

Patience and knowledge of harvest time are possessed to the "Nth" degree by Indians. Starvation and need are behind their discoveries of food and medicine. One wonders by what lengthy process of elimination, cooking methods and PROPER DOSAGE were determined.

Because there was no single staple which could be leaned upon famine was never imminent, and plant life furnished food, independent of animal life.

Discussion of old-time customs brought back an earlier and better day, when the Indian was self-sustaining, and less dependent on foods and medicines of the white man.

No strict rule was adhered to regarding medical knowledge. It was not confined to medicine men, or to the very old. Certain medicaments were spoken quietly by the older women, such as birth control remedies, or treatment for venereal diseases, but a surprising knowledge of plant uses was shown by nearly all Indian children, perhaps the Indians' natural heritage.

* * *

COLDS

BALSAM FIR (*Abies lasiocarpa*), "Wungobe," Shoshone, tea from needles and resinous blisters, at Owyhee, Nevada, and in Montana.

BUCKWHEAT, WILD (*Eriogonum umbellatum*), "Naka-donup," tea from roots for colds, Nevada.

CORAL ROOT (*Corallorhiza maculata*), no Indian name; at Owyhee and Pyramid Lake, Nevada, whole plant is dried and tea is made of bits. Same is true of Snow plant, both thought of supernatural origin.

CREOSOTE BUSH, (*Larrea tridentata*), "Ya-Temp," tea from leaves at Moapa, Nevada. Also called "Geroop" by other Paiutes.

BLUE GILIA (*Gilia spp.*), "Aqui he binga," tea from whole plant for children, Austin and Ely, Nevada Shoshones.

GUM PLANT, (*Grindelia squarrosa*), "Sanaka para," Shoshone, Cough medicine, upper third of plant dried, especially the sticky buds. "Aks-Peis," Blackfeet.

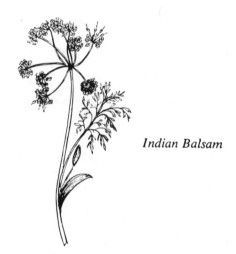

Indian Balsam

INDIAN BALSAM (*Leptotaenia multifida*), "Toza," Paiute and Shoshone, "Doza," Washoe, "Cha luksch," Warm Springs, Oregon. Tea made for coughs flu from chips. This is the BIG MEDICINE in Inter-Mountain area and in Pacific Northwest.

MEADOW RUE, (*Thalictrum species*), "Taba emlu," Washoe. Tea from root for colds.

MINT, HORSE (*Monarda species*), "Toya bawana," Bannock, Idaho, tea from seed heads for colds and as appetizer.

MOUNTAIN BALM (*Eriodictyon Californica*), Yerba Santa. Pomo Indians in California use the gummy leaf in tea for coughs, an expectorant.

MOUNTAIN MAHOGANY (*Cercocarpus ledifolius*). Bark tea for cold used by Moapa Paiutes, "Dunumbe." Pyramid Lake for bad lungs peel outer bark but leave second skin on, scrape off carefully and let it dry. Sift and when needed, boil it down and drink. Called "Toobe."

PAROSELA. Citrus plant. Tea from whole plant for colds, called "Ma good te hoo," Paiute and Shoshone. Washoes obtain this from Pyramid Lake, Nevada. Call it "Tsoho mozick." Use only straight stems for tea.

PEONY, WILD (*Paeonia Brownii*), Tea from roots for lung trouble. "Batipi," N. Paiute; "Doo yah gum hoo," Washoes; "Newatama," Paiute

RAMONA. LITTLE CHIA (*Ramona incana*), "Tube sigino," Pyramid Lake Paiutes steep leaves and give hot for colds and sore throat in children.

SAGE, MOUNTAIN BALL SAGE (*Artemisia frigida*), "Ninny kaksa miss," Blackfeet. Tea from leaves for coughs; "Na ko ha sait," Arapaho.

SNEEZEWEED, (*Helenium Hoopseii*), Blossoms crushed and used as inhalant for hay fever.

SWEET ANISE (*Osmorrhiza occidentalis*), "Bossowey," Shoshones in Smoky Valley make tea from aromatic roots with Indian Balsam, "Toza" for heavy colds and pneumonia.

WILD PEACH (*Prunus Andersoni*), "Tsanavi," Paiutes make tea from the branches for colds.

WILD ROSE (*Rosacae species*). Generally used tea from roots for colds.

YERBA MANSA, (*Anemopsis Californica*), Lizard Tail, called "Ch'-ponip" at Moapa, but "Nupitchi" at Beatty, Nevada. Tea from plant for cold.

SORE THROAT

BITTER ROOT (*Lewisia rediviva*), "Ax six sixie," Blackfeet. Pound dry root and chew it for sore throat. Old peoples' remedy. Pounded for medicine, general alterative, Fort MacDermitt, Nevada.

BLADDER POD, DOUBLE (*Physaria didymocarpa*), "Pa ki to ki," Blackfeet remedy for sore throat and stomach trouble. Gray leaves steeped.

LICORICE ROOT, (*Glycyrrhiza lepidota*), "Quitchemboo," Bannock. Root chewed for strong throat for singing; boiled for tonic.

PINYON PITCH, chewed for sore throat, resin blisters on bark best, Death Valley Shoshones.

STRING PLANT (*Psoralea lanceolata*), "Pooy sonib," Paiute name. Arapahos chew fresh leaves for throat and voice.

RATTLE WEED (*Aragallus lagopus*), Purple Loco. "A sat chiot ake," Blackfeet. Chewed for sore throats and to allay swellings.

BLOOD COAGULATOR

STARRY SOLOMON'S SEAL (*Smilacina stellata*), "Wambona." The slender round root is gathered in the Fall, and dried, after cutting it cross-ways, in little rings. It is then threaded and hung up, so when a wound will not stop bleeding, this root is pounded into powder and thrown on it. Blood clots almost immediately.

EYES

ALUM ROOT (*Heuchera glabella*), "Apos i poco," Blackfeet. Root steeped for eye-wash. Also (*Heuchera parvifolia*).

ACACIA, "Pah oh pimb," Moapa Paiutes. For inflammation of eyes, due to dust, vaqueros or travelers habitually carry acacia seeds and put four in each eye on retiring.

FLAX, BLUE (*Linum Lewisii*), "Poohi natesua," Shoshone. Root steeped for eye medicine.

PINK PLUMES (*Sieversia ciliata*), "So yaits," Blackfeet. Root boiled and applied to eyes.

SANDWORT, (*Arenaria sp.* probably *rosea*). Roots for eye-wash, tea. Beatty.

SPURGE (*Euphorbia arenicola*), "Tubicai," Moapa Paitues. Lacy green mat clinging to gravelbars. Tea from whole plant for eyewash.

TURTLE-BACK (*Psathyrotes ramosissima*), "Sebu mogoonobu." This is also called Toothache plant. Tea from leaves only for eye-wash.

Special Paiute remedies: At Fort MacDermitt tea from leaves of little sagebrush was used to wash out eyes. Old blades of rye-grass, were used to scrape the eyelids, "Pohekwahane." This was part of the old treatment for trachoma. Pyramid Lake people used tea from second bark of mountain mahogany. Bark dried and sifted first.

Burns Band of Paiutes at Owyhee, used leaves of pink and white pent-stemon and leaves of Stansbury phlox for eye-wash. Tea from bark of antelope brush to clear pus from the eyes. Seeds of wild peony, "Bati pava" crushed raw and soaked in water for eye medicine. Flaxroot tea, as a wash, with poultices of Poverty weed, "Durunzip" for severe cases.

Shoshones in Ruby Valley cut fresh root of Indian Balsam (*Leptotaenia multifida*), "Toza" and collect the drops of oil which come out. One drop of this is put in each eye of a trachoma sufferer. Said to be positive cure with one application.

FEVER

CLEOME, YELLOW. BEE PLANT (*Cleome surrulata*), "Pokusinop," Warm Springs, Oregon, uses whole plant for tea for fever.

CLEMATIS, WHITE (*Clematis ligusticifolia*), "Tum kicks kola," Warm Springs, Oregon, steeps white portion of bark for fever.

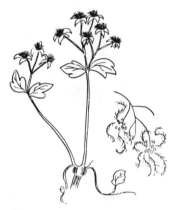

Wild Clematis

BRIDES BOUQUET (*Chaenactis stevioides*), tea to slow down heart-beats if a child has fever, used at Elko, Nevada.

HEART AND TONIC

CACTUS (*Cereus Greggii*), South of Beatty, Nevada. Root tea given as cardiac stimulant. Called there "Pain in the heart."

PINK ROOT (*Horkelia Gordonii*), Tea from root used as a tonic by the Arapahos. Root dug just before maturity has pink sap.

INDIAN BALSAM, "Toza," this is one of the most widely used midicinal plants in the Inter-Mountain area. The roots are dug after seed is ripe. They are like small carrots and have a celery fragrance. The roots are cut into dollars and strung on a line to cure in the shade. Tea is made from chips and part of the up-building is to stay in bed, and drink only "Toza" for liquid, for a week.

DOGWOOD, OSIER (*Cornus stolonifera*), inner bark has properties of quinine used as tea internally.

MOUNTAIN BALM (*Ceanothus velutinus*), "Moon-num Moon-num," Warm Springs Indians make a diagnostic tea from leaves for puzzling illnesses. The patient breathes out a fresh odor. Other names are "Snow-brush" and at Fallon, Nevada, "Sheep-herder tea," "Datzip."

WORMWOOD (*Artemisia heterophylla*), "Kose-wiup," Paiute. At Owyhee, Nevada, a basket was used to steep wormwood leaves in, and put them next to a baby's skin to reduce fever.

KIDNEY AND BLADDER TROUBLE

At Beatty, Moapa, and other desert areas where great heat, scarce, and impure water prevail, as might be expected, prominent plant remedies are for the relief of kidney and bladder troubles.

FIDDLENECK, WHITE (*Heliotropium oculatum*), Chinese pusley. "Tumanabe" called at Schurz. Whole plant tea used as emetic.

IRIS, FLAG (*Iris Missouriensis*), "Poku erop," Paiute. "Daw see doya," Shoshone. Tea from root for kidney trouble, Fort MacDermitt.

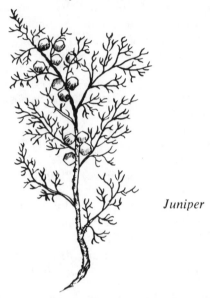

Juniper

JUNIPER BERRIES (*Juniper utahensis*), "Sammapo," Shoshone.

LUPINES, "Kamo sigi," Paiute; "Cupi chuk," Shoshone; "Wapeayta," Warm Spr. Tea from seeds at Beatty helps failure to urinate.

PENNYROYAL, TULE MINT (*Mentha arvensis*). California Indians use tea from leaves gathered when plant is in seed, for kidney complaint.

SAGE, BUD (*Artemisia spinescens*), "Kube," Fort MacDermitt Paiutes cook the plant and use juice as medicine for bladder.

SAND VERBENA (*Abronia villosa*), "Ayaho," Moapa Paiutes, inducer of urine.

TURTLEBACK (*Psathyrotes ramosissima*), "Sebu mogoonobu," Kidney and bladder.

WILD CUCUMBER (*Echinocystis spp.*). Roasted seeds eaten for kidney troubles. California Indians.

LAXATIVE, PHYSIC AND DYSENTERY

ANISE, SWEET, (*Osmorrhiza occidentalis*) "Bossowep," "Pasowoip," Shoshone. Tea from roots general physic. Antelope brush "Hunabe," leaves chewed raw for physic. For small pox, handful of leaves boiled in water to cover.

ASTER, DWARF PURPLE, "Dumbassop," Paiute; "Stop," Shoshone. Tea from cured roots for diarrhea. Same for wild buckwheat, "Segwebee."

CASCARA. COFFEE BERRY (*Cascara sagrada*), "Ae buck oko," Warm Springs, Ore. California Indians also. Bark used for physic, peeled towards ground.

CINQUEFOIL (*Potentilla Spp*), used for laxative by Paiutes. Cook whole plant which looks silvery and silky.

CHOKECHERRY (*Prunus demissa*), dried cherries pounded, mixed with dry salmon and sugar, for dysentery. Oregon Indians.

LOBELIA. Tea, emetic and physic. Shoshone.

OREGON GRAPE (*Berberis repens*), "Sogo tiembuh," Shoshone; "Kawdanup," Paiute "ch cow cow," Warm Springs; "Oti to que," Blackfeet. Root peeled, dried and steeped to check rectal hemorrhage and dysentery.

SEA HOLLY (*Eryngium alismaefolium*), "Momono Kaiyu," Paiute, Steep whole plant for diarrhea. Tiny plant 2 inches high, rare.

POVERTY WEED, (*Iva axillaris*), "Durunzip" Shoshone. For bowel disorders root soaked in cold water for tea.

SAGE, SMALL, (*Artemisia spp.*), 'Pava hobe," Paiute. Tea for physic, also

SAGE, BLACK, (*Artemisia nova*), "Bahabe," Smoky Valley, same use.

SAND DOCK (*Rumex venosus*), "Tua ono gibu," also "Tuha konobe," Shoshone. Boil whole plant for physic. In ten minutes help inside pain.

THISTLE POPPY (*Argemone hispida*), "Ishub goofwa," Paiute; "Tsagida," Shoshone, Seed tea used as physic.

WILLOW, GRAY, (*Salix exigua*), "Kosi tsube," Paiute and Shoshone. Put willow twigs in tomato can, teaspoon salt, fill up with water. Steep and drink for laxative.

Tea from leaves of Trumpet phlox, silver sage, pentstemon, stone seed, white rabbit brush, "Soana tesua," Shoshone, for general laxative.

POULTICES

For dropsy or The Swells:

BALLHEAD SANDWORT (*Arenaria congesta*) called "Hooni" or "Hoona" by Shoshones, and "Wemsee" by Washoes, who apply poultices of steeped leaves to swellings, used hot, patient lies down, as movement may bring on nosebleed.

ELDERBERRY, (*Sambucus glauca*), also the red one, (*Samb. racemosa*), "Koonogibu," Paiute; "Duhiembuh," Shoshone; Roots boiled till soft apply to caked breast or any inflammation.

JOINT GRASS, or BULRUSH, poultice from this, stems bruised for poultice for blood poisoning, by Chippewas.

DEATH CAMAS (*Zygadenus spp*), "Dabi segaw," Shoshone; "E cramps," Blackfeet. Raw roots mashed and applied for swelled knee or legache. Will adhere without bandage.

DESERT MALLOW, WILD GERANIUM, (*Sphaeralcea ambigua*), "Numanaka," Shoshone. Root cooked and applied inside of cloth for poultice. Also raw root mashed and applied to swelled feet.

WILD CURRANT (*Ribes aureum*), "Bogumbe." At Owyhee, Shoshones grind second bark for poultice. When skin turns yellow it is strong enough. Same method used for Wild Rose inner bark. Fresh rose galls mashed and applied to boils after opening, called "Tsia buwi," Paiute.

YARROW (*Achillea lanulosa*) "Pannonzia," Shoshone. Whole plant boiled and applied as poultice for felon.

WOUNDS

PLANTAIN (*Plantago major*), "Woodie," Smoky Valley Shoshones. Tea from whole plant and poultices of same for battle bruises. Also raw leaves with those of wild clematis, and apply to wounds.

ROPER'S RELIEF, YELLOW MONKEY FLOWER, (*Mimulus guttatus*), Paiute name, "Pah what na abe"; "Unda vich quana," Shoshone. Raw leaves and stems applied to rope burns on Indian vaqueros' hands.

RHEUMATISM

JUNIPER, (*Juniperus spp*), "Wapi," Paiute; "Sammabe," Shoshone; "Paal," Washo . Burn fire down to coals. Put on green juniper boughs, and have patient lie down on them and steam, drinking meanwhile tea from leaves.

PASQUE FLOWER (*Pulsatilla spp*), "Napi," Blackfeet. Leaves poultice counter-irritant for rheumatism.

PEPPERWOOD, CALIFORNIA BAY, (*Umbellularia Californica*). Crushed leaves bound on to cure headache. Leaves put in hot water, used for bathing rheumatic patients. Used in California by Yuki tribe.

SAGEBRUSH, WORMWOOD, (*Artemisia heterophylla*), "Pava hobe," Shoshone. "Poonkinny," California Indians. Packets of steamed plants placed on limbs for rheumatism, and sweat bath given.

SUNFLOWER (*Wyethia longicaulis*). Root baked, poultices for rheumatism.

For battle bruises, badger oil is well rubbed on. A psychological value to this, the badger being notably strong and courageous for his size.

WILD ROSE, "Yano," Arapaho. Both barks used for tea, beverage and medicinal. Seed cooked for muscular pains. "Stappah," berries. W. Spr.

SMALLPOX

Burn Antelope brush, juniper or Parosela on top of stove. Disinfect everything in this smoke. Drink tea from leaves and wash with it.

GUM PLANT (*Grindelia squarrosa serrulata*), "Sanaka Para," Shoshone. Upper third of plant dried, especially sticky buds, and taken for dropsy and smallpox.

SORES AND BOILS

ALUM ROOT (*Heuchera parvifolia*) "Apos—Ipoco,"Blackfeet. Root pounded up and used wet to apply to sores and swellings.

DOCK, YELLOW ROOT, (*Rumex crispus*), "Pawia"; "Matoa koa ksi," Blackfeet. Root mashed into pulp and applied to sores and swellings.

FOUR O'CLOCK (*Hesperonio retrorsa*), "Hewovey," "Paiute; "Pano-samobe," Shoshone. For sores, dry root on sun, grind fine. Peel scab, blow powder on. Known to U.S.I.S. Field nurses as Impetigo plant.

HONEYSUCKLE, (*Lonicera interrupta*). Leaves used by Yuki (California) to wash for sores. Shoshones pound raw root and apply to swellings.

HORSE-TAIL (*Equisetum arvense*), joint grass. Dried and burned and ashes used on sore mouths.

Pentstemon breviflorus, "Yaha tesa," Paiute, Fort Mac Dermitt. Leaves dry ground and used on running sores.

Pentstemon deustus, white. "Sebu," Shoshone. Root powdered, put on sores.

PHLOX, STANSBURY, (*Phlox longifolia*) "Saga donzia," Shoshone. Boiled leaves applied to boils.

PRIMROSE, ALKALI LILY, (*Pachylophus caespitosus*), "Oks pi poku," Blackfeet. Root which grows in alkali soil, pounded up and applied wet to sores and to reduce inflammation.

Pine gum applied to boils. (*Pinus edulis*), "Tuba."

SAND DOCK (*Rumex hymenosepalus*), "Big Hewovey," Paiute. Root dried powdered, used on sores and burns. "Ha ne sae huit," Arapaho. Stems and leaves used as wash for sores.

THISTLE POPPY (*Argemone hispida*), "Ishub goofwa," Paiute. Seed ground and applied to sores.

WOLF MOSS (*Evernia vulpina*). Used in California by Yukis and Wailakis for drying up running sores. Thick decoction.

STOMACH TROUBLE AND EMETICS

FLAX, BLUE, (*Linum Lewisii*) "Alai natesua," Paiute. Whole stem steeped and used for disordered stomach and gas.

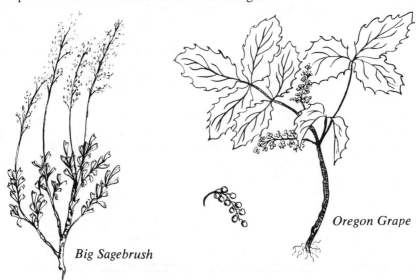

Big Sagebrush

Oregon Grape

— 44 —

OREGON GRAPE (*Berberis repens*), "O ti toque," Blackfeet. Roots boiled for stomach trouble and hemorrhages.

PEPPERMINT, (*Mentha penardi*), "Paquanah," Paiute and Shoshone. Tea from leaves and stems after drying, for gas pains.

SAGEBRUSH, BIG, (*Artemisia tridentata*), "Sawabe" Paiute and Shoshone. Leaves chewed to relieve indigestion.

VALERIAN (*Valeriana septentrionalis*), hot drink from roots for stomach trouble. Blackfeet.

YARROW, (*Achillea lanulosa*), "Pannonzia," Shoshone. Tea from root for gas pains at Owyhee, Nevada.

FOR HICCOUGHS: At Elko, tea from valerian root, "Gubeshumb," Shoshone, At Austin, tea from juniper berries, "Sammapo," Shoshone.

EMETICS

There were comparatively few remedies for indigestion. Fasting and emetics were relied upon. For poisoning, emetics were the sole reliance. All tribes used tea from ripe unground seeds of antelope brush. Tea from roots of Balsamroot, Death Camas, Wild Celery and False Hellebore was universally used.

DEATH CAMAS, (*Zygadenus spp*), "Dabi segaw," Shoshone; "Kogi a donup," Paiute; "A la pish esh," Warm Springs, Ore.; "Kogi desme," Washoe; "E cramps," Blackfeet.

LIVER

GUM PLANT (*Grindelia squarrosa serrulata*), "Aks peis," Blackfeet. Root boiled and tea taken internally.

TOOTHACHE

IRIS (*Iris Missouriensis*), "Poku erop," Paiute; "Pah sa gida," Shoshone. Root inserted in cavity will kill nerve, tooth will come out.

POPPY, CALIFORNIA (*Escholtzia Californica*), Leaves for toothache used by California Indians.

TURTLE BACK (*Psathyrotes ramosissima*), "Sebu mogoonobu." Paiute. This is called the Toothache plant in desert sections. It is called Turtle back because of its mounded shape. It is pulled up by the roots and hung up to dry. When toothache comes, dry bits are chewed on the side where the toothache is.

YARROW (*Achillea lanulosa*), "Pannonzia," Shoshone; "Todzi tonega," Paiute; "Kannam nam stuck," Wasco, Oregon; "Wapun wapun," Warm Springs, Oregon. Bit of root inserted in hollow tooth for toothache.

Hot applications of leaves, flowers and pounded root used for earache at Beatty, Nevada, called there "Wiutu."

WOMEN'S AILMENTS

CREOSOTE LEAVES (*Covillea tridentata*), "Ya temp," Moapa; "Ya tombe," DVSh. "Geroop," Paiute. Leaves steeped to relieve cramps or for irregularities.

PENNYROYAL, (*Monarda odoratissima*), "Guy mohpu," tea from flowerheads steeped for regulator for young girls.

SOLOMONS SEAL, (*Smilacina amplexicaulis*), "Shapui," Paiute; "Roy," Sho. Tea from roots for female trouble and internal pains.

TANSY, (*Tanacetum crispum vulgare*), not native. Tea from fresh leaves for suppressed menstruation, commonly used by white settlers above Smoky Valley, and brought in by Indians as a borrowed medicine.

WOMAN MEDICINE (*Porophyllum leucospermum*), "Paguidobe," Moapa. This has no common name. Regulates delayed menstruation.

WORMWOOD, SMALL SAGEBRUSH (*Artemesia gnaphalodes*), "Kose wiup," Paiute; "Pava hobe," Shoshone, "Ba wa zip," young people's tea. Smoky Valley Tea and steam bath for young girls approaching maturity.

BIRTH CONTROL

At Elko, Nevada, when the baby is one month old, a trench is filled with warm ashes. The mother lies down in them, meanwhile drinking tea from boiled root of Desert mallow, wild geranium, (*Sphaeralcea ambigua*), "Numa naka," Shoshone. Said to be safe from pregnancy until the baby is a year old.

At Beowawe, daily use of tea made from fresh root of False Hellebore (*Veratrum Californica*), "Tobassop," "Wundavassop," Sho.; "Baduppa," Washoe. Tea from cured root of same ensures sterility for life.

STONE SEED, PLANTE AUX PERLES (*Lithospermum ruderale*), "Not misha," at Owyhee. Handful of dried root, chipped, boiled in water to cover, and tea used daily for six months, results in permanent birth control.

JUNIPER BERRIES (*Juniperus spp.*), "Sammapo," Shoshone. Tea from berries taken on 3 successive days, a cupful each time, said to be efficacious.

WARTS OR MOLES:

To remove these, cut in all directions, and rub in the fuzz from prickly pear cactus, "Wogaybe"; guaranteed not to return.

SPLINTS: The most satisfactory splint for an animal's or a child's bones are made from the skin of the larger of the two Chacuala lizards which are found in extreme southern Nevada, and in Death Valley. An opportunity to bag one is never lost. The lizard is carefully skinned and the skin divided into strips which are rolled smoothly bandage fashion, and kept for emergency use. Broken bones are set and snugly wrapped with three strips of Chacuala skin, which overlap like shingles. A cloth bandage covers all. Leave till the moon is the same and ten days more.

The meat of the lizard is jerked and saved. Applied as a poultice to blood poisoning or persistent sores, with good results, as the poison is drawn to the top of the wound, while new skin forms beneath.

ODDS AND ENDS

FITS:

At Beatty, Nevada, there is a plant called Yerba Mansa, also called Lizard Tail from the shape of the flower stalk. It is also called Yerba del pasmo, because it is good for fits. Tea from the whole plnt. Called "Ch'-ponip" at Las Vegas. (*Anemopsis Californica.*)

HAIR:

Powdered root of Four o'clock (*Hesperonia retrorsa*), used as a shampoo, and tea taken inwardly at same time. Paiute name: "Hewovey."

CLEMATIS (*Clematis ligusticifolia*), "Tum kicks kola," Warm Springs. Leaves and bark used as soap and shampoo. Fort MacDermitt uses root dry and powdered for shampoo. Soap root, Yucca.

SNAKE BITE:

Fort MacDermitt advises "If a rattler bites you on the limb make a twist of horsehair above the bite, and bind mashed raw root of wild parsnip, "Hakinop" on the wound. It will draw out poison.

Elko Shoshones mash raw root of Wild Corn, False Hellebore, "Wunda vassop" on the wound, and renew when it dries out.

Juice of milkweed and tea from leaves of creosote bush are also used as poultices to draw out poison.

In northern California Indians use poultices of fresh leaves of Mexican milkweed, *Asclepias mexicana,* for snakebite.

VENEREAL DISEASES

Each group of Indians has its favorite medicine, the BIG MEDICINE, which is frequently shared with other tribes. They are used to covering great distances, and are constantly visiting and interchanging herbs, seeds and basket materials.

In Nevada, in Shoshone territory, from Elko north to Owyhee, and south to Ely, Austin and Tonopah, definite recognition is made of blood disease and the need for treatment. Throughout this country a plant tentatively identified as Ballhead Sandwort, known as "Hooni" from Elko north, and at Austin and Tonopah as "Bi Heva," is commonly used to cure gonorrhea. This is also known and used at Moapa. It is a perennial. At Charleston, on porphyry soil, the flower is red, elsewhere, it is white. It blooms and should be gathered and dried in May and June. After Fall rain it has a second blooming.

The patient prepares to be in bed three days, during which time by continuous drink of tea, hot, from whole plant, it is hoped to bring on a high fever. At Moapa, twigs of Indian Tea, Brigham, or Mormon tea, are added to the tea.

For gonorrheal ulcers, poultices of steeped leaves and blossoms of "Bi Heva" are efficacious, together with exposure to sunshine at short intervals. Scientific name of "Bi Heva" (*Arenaria congesta*).

Fort MacDermitt uses "Toza," Indian balsam, root boiled with yarrow leaves for tea. Smoky Valley has a dwarf pentstemon, "Dimbashego," whose leaves are mashed raw, and juice is used as a wash. *Pentstemon deustus.*

Roots of wild iris are boiled, tea drink, positive cure for V.D. At Las Vegas and Moapa, juniper roots, "Ah wapi" and a white root which has a yellow flower, are boiled for tea for gonorrhea. At Moapa tea from a wild melon, Buffalo gourd, (*Cucurbita foetidissima*), "Arnoko" cures gonorrhea, while the same plant called "Poonono" at Beatty cures syphilis.

Reese River, Nevada, for syphilis uses dried twigs of Ephedra, mixed with bark of antelope brush, "Hunabe" for tea.

A dwarf yellow aster, (*Erigeron concinnus*), "Ah gwe shuh" at Owyhee, is respected as a cure for gonorrhea. Tea from whole plant.

Elko used tea from roots of Meadow rue, Thalictrum species, not too strong will cure venereal diseases.

From Battle Mountain south, Trumpet phlox is extensively used. The whole plant, including flowers is steeped at Ely, Elko, Reese River Smoky Valley and Tonopah. It is a BIG Paiute remedy for blood disease though it is in Shoshone territory, and is plentiful enough to have a postoffice named after it: "Tem Paiute." Its flowers are scarlet or pink trumpets on either side of a long stem. It is also called "Sky Rocket." This plant is a biennial. Self seeds well. Worthy of a place in any garden.

Its great value is as a blood purifier, and cure for gonorrhea. Botanical name is Gilia aggregata. It is used by Shoshones freely, but they refused to talk about it, saying it was unmannerly to talk about another tribe's medicine.

A patient receiving treatment prepares to be in bed at least five days, and must not move hand or foot during that time. All available bedclothes are used. Quantities of "Tem Paiute" are steeped, and no other liquids are given the patient. This raises the fever and bedclothing helps maintain it.

HORSE MEDICINE

The horse altered the life of the Indian materially but they had very crude and tough saddles, frequently used without blankets, which started saddle sores. Many plants dried up these sores and toughened the hide, for other ailments plants were used.

MELON, WILD (*Cucurbita foetidissima*) "Arnoko," Moapa. Tea from this for bloat, also for worms.

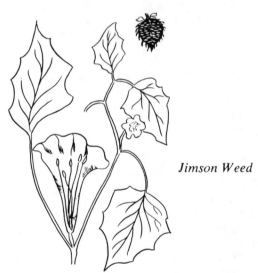

Jimson Weed

JIMSON WEED (*Datura meteloides*), "Moip," "Toloache." Tea from this to wash horse with when he wants to stray.

INDIAN BALSAM (*Leptotaenia multifida*), "Toza." In Nevada for distemper chips of "Toza" are put on slow coals on a shovel, and the horse's head covered with a sack which includes the shovel. This causes him to cough and break up his head trouble. Ground chips are also powdered fine and put on saddle sores.

FALSE HELLEBORE, (*Veratrum spp.*), "Tobassop," Shoshone. Large raw root mashed and applied to snake bite on man or beast.

ALUM ROOT (*Heuchera glabella*), "Apos-ipoco," Blackfeet. Same as preceding.

MILKWEED, (*Asclepias cryptoceras*) "Banumb," Shoshone. Juice for horses sore back.

DOCK (*Rumex crispus*), Yellow root, "Pawia." Root pounded to a pulp applied to saddle sores, Smoky Valley, Nevada.

PINE DROPS (*Pterospora andromedea*). Whole plant mashed and put on horse's sore back.

YARROW (*Achillea lanulosa*), "Pannonzia," Shoshone; "Todzi-tonega," Paiute. Leaves boiled and applied for collar boils on a horse, Ft. MacDermitt.

WILD CLEMATIS, infusion of leaves, used for cuts on horses.

FOR TONIC

SWEET CICELY (*Washingtonia divaricata*), "Paoh-coi-au-saukas," Blackfeet. "Smell mouth." Roots placed in mares' mouth, and made to chew them. Drinks more water, and put them in good condition for foaling.

Nez Perce Indians said to be the finest light cavalry in the world at the time of Chief Joseph, were very horse-conscious, and lost no opportunity to improve horse-racing. The seeds of wild peony were chewed and then put in the horse's mouth an instant before the race began. He always won. "Olap'cut Olap'cut" was Nez Perce name. "Batipi," N. Paiute. Root of wild clematis, "Tum kicks kola" was similarly used in Oregon.

TICK MEDICINE

The root of Indian Balsam made into a wash was used in Oregon to free horse from ticks; also for dandruff. "Cha luksch," Wm. Spr. This is *Leptotaenia multifida*.

CEREMONIALS AND MAGIC

ANGELICA (*Angelica Breweri*)—Magic. Root used as gambling talisman.

BEAR CURRANT (*Ribes cereum*). "Dembogem," Shoshone, Tonopah; "Tsapuwi" P.; "Skee yap" Warm Springs, Ore. These sticky currants are emetic, if too many are eaten. The bear thus reserved them for his own use.

CEDAR. Boughs on tepee poles said to ward off lightning. Thunderbird said to nest in mountain cedars. Red cedar, (*J. scopulorum*), used ceremonially on altar of the sacred woman at the Sun Dance.

GOURDS. (*Cucurbita foetidissima*), "Arnoko" Moapa; "Poonono," Shosh.

This cure-all is treated ceremonially. It is known to have both male and female flowers. For treatment the part of the plant which corresponds to the part of the body. Root for foot. Top for head.

JUNIPER (*J. Sibirica*)—The prickly one. "Bat-they-naw," Arapaho. Needles ground for scent and to drive smallpox away, thrown on hot stove or rocks. In Indian folk lore, among Shoshones, Coyote said he could make pine nuts, because he was the smartest animal, but when all gathered to watch him, they turned out to be juniper berries, "Sammapo."

ANTELOPE BRUSH (*Purshia tridentata*), "Hunabe." This with juniper and parosela, "Ma-good-te-hoo," were burned to drive the devil away in time of epidemic.

INDIAN RHUBARB (*Heracleum lanatum*), "Po-kint-somo," Bft. A stalk of this placed on altar of Sun Dance ceremonial.

INDIAN TURNIP (*Lithospermum linearifolium*), "Mass" Bft. Tops dried and burned ceremonially.

INDIAN PAINT BRUSH (*Castilleja spp*), because it is always found near rocks where rattlesnakes may lurk, is known as Snake's friend, "Taqua-qinnop"; Snake's matches, "Doo wan dayem," for decoration only. Tea from flowers for Love medicine. The rattlesnake distills poison from this flower. It is put into a love charm. Owyhee, Nevada.

DATURA, Jimson weed (*Datura meteloides*), "Moip," Moapa. This has a heavy root, which is soaked, ground and boiled. Tea renders the drinker unconscious. He will have visions, but should be watched lest he wander off in search of some lost article.

Gamblers keep root in pocket, and eat seeds while gambling. This enables them to become clairvoyant and guess correctly in hand games.

It is said that Zunis use a decoction for anesthetic.

YELLOW EVENING PRIMROSE (*Oenothera Hookeri*), "Koatsa dabe buha," Paiute Bannocks at Fort Hall, Idaho, call it "Toya notz worda," war poison. This plant grows high on the mountain. A light burns by it at night. It is a hunting charm, if it is rubbed on a hunter's moccasins and on his body, it will cause deer to come to him and snakes to avoid him. When searching for this root, do not dig it at night, drive a stake by it, and get in the daytime. The light that burns by it, is caused by phosphorescence from a decaying root. Gases.

RED LARKSPUR (*Delphinium nudicaule*), Sleep root. Root has narcotic properties, which are made use of in causing an opponent to become stupid in gambling. Tea from root.

MOUNTAIN MAHOGANY (*Cercocarpus ledifolius*), "Toobe," Paiute; "Durumbe' and "Turumbe," Shoshone. This tree lives at high elevations thunder also lives there, so traveling going up high is made safer by painting with bark decoction to ensure safety against thunder. Wear a slip of bark in your hat to protect you from thunder and lightning. It will not strike you. If you have two hats, remember to change the slip of bark over.

NEBRASKA SEDGE (*Carex nebraskensis*), Cut-your-finger, "So-yo-toi-yis," Bft. Favorite food of buffalo, tied around the horns of the buffalo head in the Sun dance.

SAGE, sweet (*Artemisia dracunculoides*), "Pa-wots," Tonopah; "K'to nee" Warm Springs. "Enga pawaga" Fort Hall ceremonial plant. When dried, it has a pleasing, persistent fragrance, and is used in Sun Dance with pava hobe small sage. All sagebrush foliage considered fortunate, and formed part of the medicine man's costume among Paiutes.

SAGEBRUSH, Big, (*Artemisia tridentata*), "Sawabe" P. Washoe medicine man used this sagebrush about his costume. This is the State flower of Nevada. Sagebrush moccasins used in Nevada sun dances. Sagebrush is burned at the beginning of all ceremonies. A sinner must bathe with sagebrush. Brooms for the Sun Lodge are made of sagebrush.

CUDWEED SAGEBRUSH, Mugwort, (*Artemisia gnaphalodes*), "Kosi sawabe," P. "Pava hobe." Used in and about Sun Dance Lodge. Dancers bathe with it as they come out from the dance.

MOUNTAIN BALL SAGE (*Artemisia frigida*), "Na-ko-ha-sait," Arapaho. Whole plant used for ceremonials, by Arapaho.

PAROSELA, Desert Rue, Citrus plant, (*Parosela,* or *Dalea spp*), some species called "Ma-good-te-hoo," P&S Owyhee, a hunting talisman. This at Moapa is called "Mogurup," Desert Rue. It is used to dye basket willows yellow, but is not carried on horseback, because it will cause the horse to swell up.

SWEET GRASS (*Savastana odorata*), "Se padzimo," Bft. Has a ceremonial use. Is gathered and braided, put up in Sun Dance altars, and in any religious service.

SUNFLOWER, Balsamroot, "Ah-kerh," Paiute; (*Balsamorrhiza sagittata*). "A pono-kauki," Bft. Paper leaves. These leaves are used in camas roasting ceremonial.

"Yarrube," Magic. Mineral, probably graphite, in pockets, Bridgeport, Calif. Used in medicine man's ceremonies, rubbing on patient's body and hair.

BOWS AND ARROWS

In fairly early days in Nevada, Indians acquired guns, and learned to use them, but their cost and weight—for the old trade guns were heavy—before they had horses to carry them, kept the use of bow and arrow active long after the country was settled by the white. Another factor was the silence of the lighter weapon.

Washoes formerly used the emery-like stems of horse-tails, (*Equisetae*), "Mep," to smooth bow and arrow. They used arrow wood, (*Philadelphus spp.*) for the shafts, yew for the bows, and flint points. All of this material was obtained in the California mountains, near Lake Tahoe which area is a summer home for them. Cedar (*Librocedrus decurrens*) was also for bows.

Deer sinew was used for bowstring, with occasionally string made from wild clematis, (*Clematis ligusticifolia*). Death Valley Indians used string from Indian hemp, (*Apocynum spp.*).

Paiutes and Shoshones used juniper for bows, with a good springy willow in the mountain districts. Near Moapa, mesquite or desert willow was popular, especially from a partially dead and leaning tree.

Small bird arrows were made from the long shoots of the snowberry, (*Symphoricarpus racemosus*), "Pam bigama," Paiute, "Newa," Shoshone. This was cut down in Fall, so that it would send up shoots the following Spring and be straight and smooth by autumn. This wood is very light and has a very large pith, which can be drawn out to make an arrow of any desired weight.

Arrows for duck hunting made from the stout stalks of wild sugar cane, (*Phragmites communis*), were called "Weg-we-kobuh." These arrows were in two pieces, foreshaft of cane, "Behabe," Lovelock, and "Pahrump" Moapa, and tip of mountain mahogany, (*Cercocarpus ledifolius*), "Toobe" and "Turumbe," Shoshone, which had been fire-hardened. Near Lovelock arrow points are of flint, bound on with deer sinew.

At Moapa, the tips are of mesquite wood, fire-hardened. They are attached to the shaft with the red gum which is found on the creosote bush, (*Covillea tridentata*), "Ya-tombe." This gum is really a lac deposited by a small insect. The arrow is called "Sa-waj," and is lightly feathered with narrow feathers, paralleled, not spiralled.

At Indian Springs, between Beatty and Las Vegas, was found a reddish wedge-shaped stone, harder than sandstone, with a hole bored through it just below the wide top. It was an arrow straightener. When small wood is used for arrow-shafts, as is frequently necessary on the desert, it is sometimes crooked and cranky. It was customary to wet the wood and having heated the straightener, pass the shaft through the hole until the crooks were removed.

SYRINGA, Wild, Mock-orange, (*Philadelphus Gordonianus*). In northern California, this handsome shrub was once much used for bows and arrows. The older less pithy wood was used for bows, and the young shoots for arrows, frequently tipped with mountain mahogany, (*Cercocarpus betuloides*) in solid chunks, sharpened to a point.

OSAGE ORANGE, Bow-wood, (*Maclura aurantiaca*), also called in the middle West, "Bòdark," a corruption of French "Bois d'arc," wood for bows, valued for its extreme toughness. By pioneers of Covered wagon days it was valued for axle-trees. In California planted as a hedge and for silkworm feed from leaves. Root and bark yield a yellow dye.

Horn bows were made by the Kootenay Indians. Narrow strips of mountain sheep's horns were steamed and softened and split into layers. These are covered with others and bound with sinew. Put on wet and shrunk. Plains Indians willingly traded a good horse for a bow like this.

In California the whole skin of a badger or fox used for quiver, fur side out.

DYE PLANTS

There are on every Reservation many dye plants and shrubs. Many of these have medicinal qualities.

Dyes are needed for the following: Basketry materials, Buckskin, feathers and wool.

Some plants require a mordant and on this depends the color. For every dye plant a mordant is close at hand, whether it be another plant, or in desert regions, a mineral.

Lichens seldom need a mordant, among these are Wolf Moss, (*Evernia vulpina*), "Tama mùklth muklth," Warm Springs, Ore., or Ground Lichen (*Parmelia molluscula*); the rock lichens which yield such a fine red, also are non-fading.

MORDANTS: Native alum or alunite, found in deserts, is extensively used as a mordant, usually being roasted first. A plant with the same properties found in Plains areas is Alum root, (*Heuchera glabella*). This is also a medicine plant. Its properties are in the root. Two finger lengths of root to largest size dishpan of dye is satisfactory.

In desert sections sometimes fermentation instead of boiling is used. Long boiling may change the color originally desired, as in the case of madder, it makes a beautiful red, or if boiled too long, turns yellow.

For safe carrying dried dyes are useful. In which case, stalks, seeds roots and plants must be soaked before using at least overnight.

Commercial dyes for blanket wool, as in the case of Navajos, are not desired by traders, and purchasers of rugs. Native plant dyes have an advantage if used without mordants, in that they fade, if they fade at all, in their own color scale. Reds for instance, would fade in another shade of red, and not in a dingy brown.

Dye plants following are arranged in order of color obtained: Black: Bee Plant, Cleome, pink flowered, (*Cloeme serrulata*). Arizona and New Mexico Indians boil this plant till black and gummy. This is called "Guaco" and makes a permanent beautiful black.

BLACK: Three-lobed sumac, Squaw bush, (*Rhus trilobata*), has the following Indian names: At Moapa, called "See-a-wimb," at Warm Springs, Ore. "T'net," and by Utes called "Ish." Slender twigs of this shrub are rolled up with their leaves and used either fresh or dry. Pitch from the pinyon and yellow ochre are added and all boiled together to make the best Indian black dye.

BLUE: also VIOLET: Sandalwood, the Lost Blue of Arapahos, (*Comandra pallida*), see under Paint.

Sky Rocket, Trumpet Phlox, (*Gilia aggregata*), "Tem Paiute" has blue dye in its roots.

VIOLET: Sarvis Berry or Service Berry, violet dye from fruit.

Antelope brush, (*Purshia tridentata*), "Hunabe," gives beautiful violet color from ripe seed coats cooked.

Mountain mahogany (*Cercocarpus ledifolius*), inner bark, purple dye.

BROWN: Juniper (*Juniperus monosperma*), "Wapi," Paiute; "Sammabe," Shoshone. Bark, berries and needles used for brown-tan dye. For a mordant, use green juniper needles only and burn, save the ashes and add to dye.

— 53 —

GREEN: Mountain Ball Sage (*Artemisia frigida*), leaves only, makes a soft pretty green.

Big Sagebrush, (*Artemisia tridentata*), "Sawabe," whole plant, set with alum.

RED: *Echinodontia tinctoria,* "Conk," fungus grows in conifers makes a brilliant orange-red dye.

Fomes laricus, see Cosmetics.

Chokecherry, (*Prunus melanocarpa*), juice makes a beautiful red.

Cinquefoil, (*Potentilla spp*), Cook the whole plant which looks silvery, silky, for red dye.

Madder (*Galium boreale*) Bedstraw, beautiful red from fine roots. Especially good for wool, quills or horsehair. If boiled too long it turns yellow.

Lithospermum spp. (*Galium tinctorum*) both give red.

Mountain mahogany, (*Cercocarpus ledifolius*), Rose-red dye from nodules on the roots.

Three-lobed sumac, bark in mountain areas with leaves gives red-brown. Berries on wool gives dusty-pink. Berries mashed and fermented, not boiled.

Lichen on rocks, gives red, scrape off after rain.

YELLOW AND ORANGE: Coneflower (*Ratibida columnaris*), onion skins, the part you throw away. Oregon grape, root, yellow; Snakeweed, (*Gutierrhiza*), Osage orange, yellow dye from root; Rabbit brush, (*Chrysothamnus nauseosus*) blossoms only; Sand Dock, (*Rumex venosus*), Root peeled makes burnt orange dye; Wild Rose, yellow dye from inner bark, same for Chokecherry; Wolf moss, (evernia vulpina), being a lichen, it requires no mordant, porcupine quills placed with moss in boiling water.

Dyeing experiment with Sand Dock at Wind River, Wyo. 1/4-lb. dry roots broken into bits, soaked in 1 gal. water several days. Put on in same water. Boil in enamel kettle, 2 hrs., covered. Mash and strain, bring to a boil again. Skim and continue boiling. Add 5c worth of alum, stir till dissolved. Wet 1/2-lb. of white wool yarn, add to dye-bath. Stir occasionally. Boil another hour uncovered. Leave in dye-bath overnight. Next day rinse thoroughly, until water comes clear. Dry in shade. Color will be gold or bright orange.

Besides wool and basketry, dyes are used on buckskin and on feathers. In Montana a skin dye is made from Yellow paintbrush (*Orthocarpus luteus*), "E-si-match-sis," Bft. When the plant is in full bloom, it is wrapped up with the skin it is desired to color, the color which will be reddish-tan will draw all through it. This is also good for horsehair or feathers.

Dodder, (*Cuscuta spp*) makes a handsome dye for feathers.

CHEROKEE DYES—contributed by Mr. Wade at Cutbank School at Browning, Montana.

BLACK: Take 1 gallon of corn, the kind used for Indian bread. Mix wood ashes with it. Add 2 gal. water. Boil and skim the hulls out. Boil and skim again, and add golden seal roots. Add oak splints (for basket material) and boil color into them.

BROWN: To dye white oak splints: Take poplar sap. It is bright orange color. Boil with it, pine rosin.

RED: Take locust roots, the fence-post locust, and an equal amount of chestnut roots. Add rain water from a stump. Boil all together and add peach tree leaves.

TANNING HIDES

Hides of deer and elk are usually tanned with the hair removed. At one time the Government got a number of reindeer hides from Alaska, and gave them to Nevada Indians to tan, but the hide was too thin to stand up under Paiute methods of tanning. They were best suited for robes, chair seats, etc., where the hair is left on.

On Warm Springs Reservation in Oregon, the root of a wild carrot is used in tanning. (*Leptotaenia multifida*).

The root is chipped and put into the tub with the hide, which has had the hair removed. This root has a good deal of tannin in it, and it shrinks the hide, so that wetting it does not affect it as much as other methods. Deer or cow brains are rubbed into the hide to make it soft and pliable.

Wylackie tribe of northern California take brains and wrap up in gray moss, a gray-green lichen, (*Usnea lacunosa*), in brick form, then rub this later, crumbling into the hide.

Smoked hides are pre-shrunk by digging a smoke-hole, both ends in the ground of long curved branches, with hide stretched over the branches. Fire is built of old rotten wood, preferably juniper wood, and the hide is left until it takes on a uniform yellow color.

A very white hide is obtained by not smoking it, and by washing it repeatedly in thick suds of Ivory or Castile soap.

White hide is commonly used for women's ceremonial dresses, which are heavily beaded in bright colors. Men's costumes are frequently made from mule deer hides as they are larger and heavier. A tanned hide is called buckskin. Heavy ceremonial costumes are cleaned with a white clay found on Flathead Reservation in Montana, this clay is called gypsum. Gypsum is very popular with Rocky Mountain goats, who paw it out and eat it for its salty taste. These are the goats whose likeness may be seen on freight cars of the Great Northern Railway.

ODDS AND ENDS

BABY BEDS: Down of Cat-Tail, (*Typha latifolia*), "Tabu'Oo," Paiute; "Toiba," Washoe. Used for baby beds.

BABY POWDER: Old black leaves of sagebrush found under the bushes powdered and used for rash on babies.

COSMETICS: Conk, a fungus grows in conifers (*Fomes laricus*), on Douglas fir, in Oregon, where it has several Indian names, called "Coonch" and "Shuppenchush" by Warm Springs Indians, "Nookt-nookt" by Wascoes.

It is dried, roasted and ground by Warm Springs, used as face cream to prevent sunburn. In early days it was called "Punk" by whites, and used for tinder with flint-lock guns. Grease is added to the face cream to make it spread. It has a beautiful red color.

INDIAN ROUGE: Snowdrops, white forgetmenots, (*Plagiobothrys campestris*). Grows profusely in gravelly soil in parts of northern California. Flowers have a vanilla fragrance. At base of the stem and about the roots, is red coloring matter, which is said to contain alkanin, which was formerly used as rouge.

TATTOOING: In northern California, tattooing was formerly quite common. The method used was to draw the design with poison oak juice on the face, then prick in soot with a sharp pointed needle from the nutmeg tree. This gave a blue-green color, unfading.

Certain marks' were tribal marks, notably three straight marks on the chin, known as 111, but individual could choose other patterns. On Hoopa reservation, chins were sometimes solidly blue.

BEADS: Juniper berries were pierced and used for beads near Ely, Nev. There, as in northern California, the sweet fruited juniper berries were used. The fresh ripe berries were scattered over the tall anthills, the busy, sweet-seeking ants ate out the sweet streak near the seed, leaving the desired perforation by which to string the beads.

Silverberries (*Eleagnus argentea*), "Napi," Blackfeet. Before the coming of the white man, Blackfeet women used the seeds of this Silverberry for necklaces. These berries look like pure silver, the outside tastes like raw potato, this is chewed off, and the seeds which look like fluted olive seeds are boiled till they can be pierced with a locust thorn, then they were threaded on sinew. Sometimes small agate beads were interspersed at intervals. During World War II every Blackfeet boy who went to war, had a rosary made of these beads.

BEVERAGES, see under Foods.

COMBS: Before the white man came, a branch of Cedar brush, (*Tetradymia glabrata*), whose twigs set at right angles to the stem, was used for combs.

CUPS: Austin Indians boiled whole plant of desert mallow or wild geranium down thick and added it to red clay to make it mold more easily into cups. (*Sphaeralcea ambigua*), "See-goina-kumbe," Shoshone.

DIAPERS: Old people at Ely told of an unusual use for the bark of antelope brush and cedar. Very old shrubs were sought with long shreds of soft bark, this was worked over by hand to remove harshness, and loosely plaited to wrap around the baby.

GUM: Following pine nut gathering pine gum is collected, from trees which were gashed during the preceding season. It is then carefully picked over and melted down, placed in the sun or over slow coals to render it soft enough to use. (Fishlake Paiutes, near Tonopah.) It is used for covering Paiute water-bottles, and medicinally for sores and on boils.

CHEWING GUM: Among Washoes the gum in hard knots on Desert Gum plant, (*Lygodesmia spp*), is collected and chewed. "Wa-ha-nane," Washoe. Lumps and knots on limbs of rabbit brush also chewed for gum, called "Baw-buh," Washoe.

Shoshones break the tall milkweed, (*Asclepias speciosa*) and collect the milk and roll it in the hand, until it becomes firm enough to chew. Tonopah and Beatty call it "Samoko."

Paiutes use gum from root of Arrow-leaved Balsamroot sunflower. This plant is called "Ah-kerh."

Mesquite gum is used to make designs on pottery. Dry gum is mixed with fat for salve on sores.

In Utah, Trumpet Phlox (*Gilia aggregata*) the whole plant is boiled for glue by Utes.

HAIR

CLEMATIS. Virgin's bower, (*Clematis ligusticifolia*), "Tum-kicks-kola," Warm Springs, Ore. Leaves and bark used as shampoo. At Fort MacDermitt, Nevada, the root is dried and powdered for shampoo.

FOUR O'CLOCK (*Hesperonia retrorsa*), powdered root used as shampoo and tea taken inwardly at the same time. Paiute name: "Hewovey."

MEADOW RUE, False Maidenhair (*Thalictrum spp*), "Taba emlu," Washoe; "Esag wena," Paiute; "Pawaga," Shoshone; "Esteewia," Warm Springs, Ore. California Indians dry the roots and use for shampoo.

SOAP ROOT (*Chlorogallum pomeridianum*), extensively used by Indians wherever it grows to wash clothes with, and as shampoo. The large bulb is divested of the coarse fibres that surround it, and the bulb is split and used as bar soap would be. Great care must be taken to rinse the hair thoroughly. It is an afternoon bloomer, hence the pomeridianum part of the name.

YUCCA: Many kinds of yucca are used for washing clothes and wool, and especially for shampoo in some Indian wedding ceremonies. Great bowls of yucca suds are prepared, and bride and groom wash each other's heads. Notably *Yucca glauca* and *Yucca baccata* are used for this.

In California the filmy flowers of the Wild lilac, (*Ceanothus spp*) any of the buckthorns, make a delightfully fragrant soapsuds.

MUSIC: Dance clappers in northern California were made of elder, and so were flutes. This was sambucus glauca.

Rattles in some parts of California were made of deer hoofs, and turtle shells. In northern California, cocoons of the California silkworm were fastened on a coyote bone, with small rocks inside, with curly feathers from a wild drake's tail in between the cocoons. This was a medicine rattle, not used for dancing.

Whistles were made from heavy reeds, and from willow in Spring. In Nevada, the red elderberry, "Koono-gibu" was used for whistles and for flutes, at Fort MacDermitt, and in the south, at Tonopah, Joint grass, horse-tail, (*Equisetum arvense*) was used for whistles, called "Mujeranga" there. Shoshone.

PERFUMES: Bed-straw, fragrant, (*Galium triflorum*) Dried flowers used to perfume belongings. This is called "Madder's Cousin."

BISCUIT-ROOT (*Cogswellia spp*), "Couse" Warm Springs, Ore. Seeds which are aromatic are carried by men for a love-charm.

MEADOW RUE (*Thalictrum spp*), Coyote angelica, "Esteewia," Warm Spr. "Pawaga," Shoshone. Seeds crushed for perfume at Owyhee, Nevada. Blackfeet and Gros Ventres dry whole plant for perfume, and put berries in buckskin bag.

PINK PLUMES (*Sieversia ciliata*) "So-yaits," Bft. Ripe seed pods crushed and used for perfume.

SWEET PINE Balsam Fir (*Abies lasiocarpa*), "Katoya." Mixed with grease to make fragrant hair-oil.

WILD CELERY, "P'tish-p'tish," Warm Springs, Oregon. Blossoms dried and used for perfume.

CATS CLAW (*Acacia Greggii*), "Bi-Joarum," Moapa. Buds and blossoms of cats claw dried and kept among women's things for sachet.

TEPEES

There is a theory that Indians were not always inhabitants of this country. One possibility considered is that they may have crossed on the ice at Bering Straits, and then scattered out, east or north or south according to their health or liking. Those who could endure hardship, or who wanted to hunt, naturally took to the Plains or to the mountains, while old or delicate Indians sought warm places where they could camp and raise part of their food. Those interested in fishing tarried by the rivers and lakes. Their homes were naturally built of materials which they found near by.

In the Southwest and in hot desert countries they found soil from which they made adobe bricks.

In Nevada tules and willows were bound together in a sort of crude weaving for "Kani," the Paiute name for summerhouse.

In the Buffalo country hides were used. This made tepees the most light, compact and portable house ever known. Buffalo hides were taken in Spring when hides and hair were thin. These were buffalo cow-hides. Lodge pole pines were used for the tripod which supported the tepee. For an average family tepee which made a room 16 feet across, it took 8 hides, with 14-16 poles to support the skins which were sewed with rawhide or sinew. There were also 2 ear-poles or dampers which controlled the smoke-hole at the top. These had flaps, and were turned according to the wind, just as a damper controls an oven.

A very large tepee intended for a council chamber might require 20 or 30 hides. A fire-pit was in the center of the tepee directly beneath the smoke-hole. A curtain of hide or later on, of canvas, ran all the way around the tepee from the floor up to about 3½ feet. This curtain kept out cold winds, dust and stray dogs. The tepee door always faced the east; as the prevailing wind blew from the west, this arrangement kept the tepee warm and comfortable. The owner sat facing the door and the place of honor was at his side. If a man had more than one wife the favorite wife sat by him. She was called The Sits-Besides-Him wife.

It was women's work to put up the tepees. At Blackfeet Reservation in Montana, every 4th of July there is still a Women's Tepee Race to see which woman can put up her tepee quickest. Race ½ mile, put up 8 poles, 10 pegs and 5 buttons.

The lodge poles are carried on a travois, and a buffalo hide served to carry the owner's belongings. The travois was composed of 2 poles attached like thills to a horse which drew it. Shallow stones acted like buttons in which were set the tepee poles to brace their huge skin house. All over the far places of the Reservation still may be found these circles of stones which show where the favorite camping places once were, always beside a clear brown stream.

The door of the tepee was closed when necessary by a skin flap. Cords on the smoke pole flaps were tied to a peg infront of the door to swing the poles around and make ventilation easy. The hide wall was also staked. It was a rule of courtesy that no one should pass between any one else and the fire.

At the sides of the tepee back-rests were arranged at the end of soft beds made of robes of buffalo or of fur animals. These backrests were made of willow rods, smooth and even, shaped like inverted wedges one half yard wide at top and a yard at bottom, they were woven together with sinew. Beds were made on small parallel logs staked down covered with pine or cedar boughs, then the robes laid over all With the back rests to support the entire back and lean the head against, this is one of the most restful couches imaginable.

On the outside of the tepee are painted various happenings in the life of the owner. Perhaps an animal which has appeared to the man in a dream, and gave him advice. This animal henceforth is the man's guardian spirit, and may be painted on his tepee, on his chest like a totem or on his shield. War tepees never registered defeat. This may have a psychological effect.

Paints used for decorating a tepee were usually of mineral origin. Some rocks were one color when collected, but after roasting would change color and would become easier to grind up in stone mortars.

Rawhide boxes were also painted in this manner with tribal patterns. These were called parfleches. Fleche being the French word for arrows, which were originally carried in these containers. These were painted among the Plains Indians with Sandalwood, (*Comandra pallida*). No true Indian name is known for this plant, but Arapahos call it "The Lost Blue," because all the Old People who knew how to use it are gone. At Uintah-Ouray information on this was that the blue dye which is beneath skin on the root was powdered, and mixed to paint thickness with juice of the round pin-cushion cactus, "Mu-zuh," Shoshone, with the liquid from an animal's eye, or with ox gall. Then it was applied to the rawhide box.

SHIELD: Among Plains Indians, a war shield was made of buffalo hide from the neck because it was thicker. When a warrior was at home, his shield was placed on an easel near his tepee, like a doorplate. When in use on horseback, the shield was slung on the underside on his left arm. This left the hands free for use of bow.

PAINT: White clay paints white without any preparation, near Tono-pah called "Ee-bee." Near Elko this called "Odumbe."

On the shores of Pyramid Lake, Nevada, in cliffs, are pockets of yellow clay, a little water is added to this clay to make dough, which is roasted a little. This is called "Oapi." When roasted under ground with a slow fire for three days, it is named "Bishapi." All of these are used for paint, decoration, war-paint and ceremonials.

A Shoshone woman living at Elko colony said that there is a rock formation, north of Battle Mountain, called "Dossowey." The original rock is very white and hard. After baking for three days, it turns to a cinnabar red, and is used for red paint.

STRING. Carrying nets for water bottles, or snares are made from fibre of wild clematis. This is sometimes used for bowstring, if sinew is not available. (*Clematis ligusticifolia*), "Esha wana," Sho.

String Plant, White alfalfa (*Psoralea lanceolata*), "Pooy sonib." Fibrous roots can be split exceptionally fine for string, nets, etc. Fragrant, will not rot in water.

(*Psoralea macrostachya*), Leather root. California tribes formerly used inner bark for thread and root fibres for bags and for rope. It was preferred to milkweed fibre on account of its whiteness and its pleasing odor.

String milkweed (*Apocynum cannabinum*), Indian hemp. Formerly used by California Indians for string. In the fall after frost comes, the outer bark will fall off, and both this and the inner bark make excellent string. It is stretched and pulled then rolled on the leg makes a handsome string about like fishline, and just as strong.

A tall and slender milkweed (*Asclepias spp*) near Yerington, Moapa, and Lovelock is similar in uses. It is called "We-ha," "Wisha," Paiute, and at Moapa, "Wee-ee-wump." In Oregon at Warm Springs, it is called "Tah-quiss." Tough inner bark retted for nets and rope.

Willow, Arroyo, (*Salix lasiolepis*), inner bark used in Spring for rope in California.

DEER ROPE. Following is from a letter from Dr. J. W. Hudson, who was desirous of obtaining a rope made from fibre of Iris Douglassii leaves. This was in northern California. The iris has threads on the outside of each leaf. These are stripped by the women wearing a long thumb nail and a musselshell over it. The leaf is caught between the nail and the shell and a long stout thread is secured. Having procured the necessary threads the men proceed to weave the ropes and accompanying nets. A deer rope is near 20 feet long with lasso at one end, and about half an inch in diameter. This loop was set over a deer trail to catch head or antlers. Within the set loop over the trail was spread a delicate network of the same material to draw in the loop. Pomo Indians called this "Ba-dik."

TOBACCO

Tobacco was sometimes the only crop that Indians with their migrations in search of food, whether game or plant food, really counted on producing. It was one of the important introductions taken back to England from the American colonies.

Over the country types of tobacco vary. In the Rocky Mountains and Plains and through Nevada and California there were the native type of tobacco, which is a Nicotiana, and then the collection of leaves and sometimes bark of other plants, also native, but carefully blended.

There are two kinds of smoking: ceremonial, as in council, and which might include preparation for training as a medicine man, and the other kind, for sociability and pleasure.

Smoking requires a pipe. The pipe still in use among Plains Indians was usually made of pipestone from the great pipestone quarries in Minnesota, dark red in color, soft when first quarried, but becoming harder with exposure to air. The pipe itself might vary in size. It was shaped like a letter L. About eight inches in length, tapering in width. The small end was three inches in length, and then rose the pipe bowl, as large around as a man's thumb, the rest of the pipe on the balance of the L was five inches long and gradually increasing in width. The pipe-stem was made of golden sumac, a sumac which used to grow close by the pipestone quarry. This stem was about 24 inches long and an inch wide, but quite thick, flat like a carpenter's pencil. This is the way the hole through the stem was made. Gathering the sumac in Spring when the sap was up in the large pith, some meat or fish was put out where blowflies could work on it. When large maggots were on the meat, the piece of sumac which had previously been put in a can of oil or bear grease, was brought in. As the large pith had taken up the oil, it was soft, and quite a bit was dug out. The maggots were then sealed up in the stem, to either eat their way through, or die. Sometimes they did both, but there was plenty of time to do it all over again, patiently, till a long perfect hole was drilled through.

On either side of this hole column holes were made and these were usually in sets of two, about six sets to the middle of the stem. Through the two holes buckskin or rawhide strings were inserted, and on them treasures of very old Hudson Bay beads, preferably blue, were tied, sometimes abalone shell pendants, and in the very middle, medicine feathers, of some bird known to bring good luck. Flicker feathers for their bright color, and eagle down, dyed red, was put on so it could float.

This was the likeness of a chief's pipe, or a medicine pipe, usually a man would have a commoner pipe, one for a quiet smoke with a friend. This might be made of soapstone, or of a black stone, which could be worked on easily.

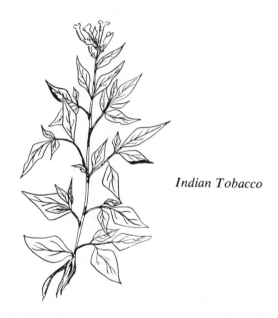

Indian Tobacco

There are different kinds of tobacco. A native tobacco, and a mixture called "Kinni-Kinnick," which is composed of leaves from the following plants and shrubs: Red dogwood, "Lotzanee," Warm Springs, Ore.; Quinine Bush, (*Garrya elliptica*); Bear berry (*Arctostaphylos uva ursi*), "Larb," "A luck," Warm Springs; "Ka sixie," also "Ka-ka-sim," Bft. Prince's Pine (*Chimaphila umbellata*), "Big Larb," "O-makse-ka-ka-sin." Both these last two from Blackfeet, who prefer "Big Larb" to all others. "Larb" is a corruption of the French term "L'herbe," of the trappers; Sandwort (*Arenaria spp*) small and silvery, its leaves were included in the mixture, called "Doomaya" by Shoshone, a term for mixture.

Nearly all these plants are found on limy soil. Creosote mistletoe in a dry form is used to add to tobacco at Moapa, where Desert Trumpet, (*Eriogonum inflatum*), "Babagorum," or swollen stalk is used as Medicine pipe. A very small pinch of tobacco being put into the wide stem. By Death Valley Shoshones, this plant is called: "Tosanan bawkip."

A natural accompaniment of the Plains medicine pipe was the tobacco bag. This was usually made of smoked buckskin with long fringes, and a six inch solid bead band at the base, beaded half inch bands on each side, and at the top in an encircling band with fringe below it. The pipe was taken apart to carry thus, and packing of moss or buffalo hair to ensure safety. The stem was also put in the bag, which had a wrist thong.

Indian tobacco, (*Nicotiana spp*), has various Indian names: Green tobacco is known as "Pwui-bamo" in Nevada, but at Beatty, "Bahombe" means cured tobacco, and may also mean cigarettes. Owyhee dries whole plant, strips slender leaves for smoking, but Battle Mountain thrashes whole plant for use, seeds and all. At Pyramid Lake, Paiute country, the whole plant is dried, and diluted with Bull Durham, or Man with coat on, Prince Albert, and "Toza," Indian Balsam chips added for a cold.

In California, a wooden pipe is made from the root of Mountain mahogany, (*Cercocarpus betuloides*), which root has an elbow used for pipe bowls. This wood is also used for digging sticks and clubs.

The local ash tree is used for pipes, according to Chesnut's book *Plants Used by Indians of Mendocino County*. "Straight pipes are made . . . out of a section of limb a foot long, and two inches thick. The bowl is dug out with a knife, and a red-hot wire is forced through the pith. As the bowl is not at an angle with the stem, it can only be used with the smoker is lying down."

Also in California, a would-be medicine man fasts for three days then smokes Indian tobacco, and watches for the dream which will come to reveal his future life. Medicine men also smoke ceremonially as a mark of respect and for curing illness.

SNUFF. White Hellebore (*Veratrum speciosum*) dry root pounded and snuffed. "Etawa-asi," Bft.

Smoking was in vogue with northwestern Indians from the time of Lewis and Clark, but they used the native mixture, kinni-kinnick. Ceremonial smoking was the same with all Indians, blowing the smoke to the four cardinal points, to the sun, and lastly to the earth. Before any important deed the pipe is smoked, for declaring of war, or ratification of peace.

An aid in making fire was the carrying of a fire-horn. This was a buffalo horn among Plains Indians. It was carefully hollowed out and lined with moist rotten wood. It had a sling to carry it by, and the tip end was plugged with a wooden cork. On top of the damp wood was placed a piece of punk, the fungus which grows in conifers, and at the beginning of a journey one coal was put on this, and the fire-horn tightly closed.

When the party arrived at camp, one person, the one who carried the fire-horn hastily started the campfire, and the women scurried around to gather wood and get the cooking fire going from the first one.

DICTIONARY OF PLANT NAMES

For the convenience of the reader plant names have been arranged in one straight catalog, dictionary form, as follows:

COMMON NAME	INDIAN NAME	BOTANICAL NAME
Alder	Psonee *WS*	Alnus tenuifolia

Because more work was done in Nevada than in any other area, more information was available on plants in that region.

Spelling of Indian names for plants is entirely phonetic, vowels are pronounced as in Italian, except that in a termination of "ai" as in "Tubicai," or "Yavapai," it is pronounced as eye.

Abbreviations for tribal names used to save space, e.g.: *Bnk*—Bannock, *Bft*—Blackfeet, *NP*—Northern Paiute, *P*—Paiute, *Pap*—Papago, *Sho*—Shoshone, *W*—Washoe, *WS*—Warm Springs, Oreg.

No official work was done in California, except at Death Valley—a short trading post project for Carson Agency. These were Panamint Shoshones, usually called Death Valley Shoshones—*DVSho*.

Mendocino County, California, has been the writer's home for fifty years but these Indians have almost entirely forsaken the old-time ways of their ancestors except for a few basket-makers near Ukiah. Practically no Indian names are available except in Chesnut's book. The Indians themselves are reluctant to recall them.

For convenience of the reader, names have been arranged in one straight alphabet. Name of the tribe will follow Indian name.

COMMON NAME	INDIAN NAME	BOTANICAL NAME
Acacia; Catclaw	Pah oh pimb; Bi-joarem Chuarem *Moapa P*	Acacia greggii
Alder	Hoowiup *Sho* Psonee *WS* A-much-ko-Iyateis *Bft*	Alnus tenuifolia
Alfalfa	Pawgeta *P* Boong go dekah *Sho*	Medicago sativa
Alum Root	Apos-ipoco *Bft*	Heuchera glabella
Angelica	Kusiginobe *Sho*	Angelica breweri
Anise; see Sweet Anise		
Ant eggs	Anino *P*	
Antelope Brush; Bitter Brush	Hunabe *P & Sho* Bal-nat-san *W*	Purshia tridentata
Arbor, summerhouse	Haba *P*	
Arrowhead; Tule Potato	Wapato *Oreg* Katniss *Algonquin*	Sagittaria latifolia
Arrow-wood; Wild Syringa		Philadelphus lewisii spp. gordonianus
Arrows	Wegwekobuh from sugarcane Sawaj *Moapa P* Kah-so *WS*	
Aspen; see Cottonwood		

—63—

COMMON NAME	INDIAN NAME	BOTANICAL NAME
Aster, Dwarf Purple	Dumbassop *P*	Erigeron spp.
	Stop *Sho*	
Aster, Dwarf Yellow	Ak-gwe-shuh *P* & *Sho*	Erigeron spp.
Atole	Aztec name for porridge of corn or seeds	
Baby Basket	Hoop *P*	
	Kono *Sho*	
	Tum-tsuss-iss *WS*	
	Loxtoo *Calif Hoopa*	
	Sekah *Ukiah·Pomo*	
Ballhead Sandwort	Bi-Heva *Sho*	Arenaria congesta
	Wemsee *W*	
	Hooni *Sho*	
Balsam Fir	Wungobe *Sho*	Abies lasiocarpa
	Katoya *Bft*	
	Tza wungobe *Ft. Hall Sho*	
Barley, Meadow	Quasi wahab *P*	Hordeum (probably) californicum
Basket, big flaring, small bottom	Ong-mo *DVSho*	
Basket, bottle-neck	Pono *DVSho*	
Basket Grass		Nolina bigelovii
Bearberry	Kinni-kinnick *Rocky Mts.*	Arctostaphylos uva-ursi
	A luck *WS*	
	Ka-sixie *Bft*	
	Larb (also refers to Prince's Pine)	
Bear Grass; or Basket Grass	Ah pay *Bft*	Xerophyllum tenax
Bedstraw, fragrant; Madder's Cousin		Galium triflorum
Bee Plant, pink	Guaco *Navajo*	Cleome serrulata
Bee Plant, yellow	Pokusinop *P*	Cleome lutea
Birch, red	Enga coniup *Sho*	Betula occidentalis
	Hoo-wee-dzup *Bnk*	
Biscuit Root	Coush *WS*	Lomatium spp. (Cogswellia group)
	Hub-hub-ma (3 finger cakes) made from Luksh (larger form) meal	
Bitterroot	Ax six sixie *Bft*	Lewisia rediviva
	Kanigda *P*	
	Pe ah ke *WS*	
	Gunga *Sho*	
Bladderpod, double	Pakitoki *Bft*	Physaria didymocarpa
Blazing Star	Ku-ha *P*	Mentzelia albicaulis & laevicaulis
Breadroot	Pomme blanche *French*	Psoralea esculenta
	Tipsinnah *Sioux*	
Bride's Bouquet		Chaenactis stevioides
Brodiaea	Winida *NP*	Brodiaea spp.
Buckeye		Aesculus californica
Buffalo	Peskan	
Buffalo Flower		Thermopsis gracilis

COMMON NAME	INDIAN NAME	BOTANICAL NAME
Bull Berries; Buffalo Berries; Silver Berries; Buck Berries	Auch ha haybena *Arapaho* Weapuwi *P* Weyumb *Sho* Me e nixen *Bft*	Shepherdia argentea
Bunch Grass	Sopeeva *P*	
Cactus	Tah-wimps *DVSho* Tu-gimb (seed)	Echinocactus polycephalus
Cactus (dried fruit)	Navoo *Sho* Ost staxie mon *Bft*	
Cactus, ladyfinger	Tsoha *Sho*	Mammillaria spp.
Cactus, night blooming	Pain-in-the-heart	Cereus Greggii ?
Cactus, round	Mu-zuh *Sho*	
Cactus, yellow flowered	Wo-waybe	
Camas, blue	Kogi *P* Pasigo *Sho* Gamooa *Wasco, Ore.* Quamash *Umatilla, Ore.* Camas *Nez Perce* Miss-iss-sah *Bft*	Camassia spp.
Camas, Death; see Death Camas		
Cascara; Coffeeberry	Ae buch oko *WS*	Rhamnus purshiana
Catclaw; see Acacia		
Cat-Tail	Tabu-oo *P* Toiba *W*	Typha latifolia
Celery, Wild	Hobe *S* Ik-nish *Klamath* Mo-zook-addas *W* P-tish-p'tish *WS* (pertains to whole plant) Cum-see (pertains to stalk below umbel)	
Chacuala lizard	Black one *Death Valley*	
Chinese Pusley; Heliotrope; Fiddleneck, white	Tumanabe	Heliotropium curassavicum var. oculatum
Choke Cherry	Daw-esha bui *P* Too-mash (the bush) *WS* Too-mish (the fruit) Tsamchit *W*	Prunus spp.
Cinquefoil, silvery		Potentilla spp.
Clematis; Virgin's Bower	Tum kicks kola *WS* Esha wana *Sho*	Clematis ligusticifolia
Cleome; see Bee Plant		
Cliff Rose; Signal Plant		Cowania mexicana var. stansburiana
Coffeeberry; see Cascara		
Columbine	Puh wha na habu *P*	Aquilegia spp.
Compass Plant	Wodzi-kuh *NP*	Euphorbia lathrys
Coral Root		Corallorhiza maculata
Cottonwood	Sohobe (pointed leaf) Singabe *Sm. V. Sho* Sawhabe	Populus trichocarpa
Cottonwood; Aspen	Sinnabe	Populus tremuloides

COMMON NAME	INDIAN NAME	BOTANICAL NAME
Creosote Bush	Ya tombe or Ya-temp *Moapa P*	Larrea tridentata
	Geroop *P*	
Currant, Bear or Wax	Skee-yap *WS*	Ribes cereum
	Tsapuwi *P*	
	Wood un de kan *Sho*	
	Dembogen *Sho Tonopah*	
Currant, Black	Owa pawump *Ft. Hall Sho*	
Currant, Wild Golden	Bogumbe *P & Sho*	Ribes aureum
	Pokops *P*	
	Mobabuwi *Yerington P*	
Death Camas	Dabi segaw *Sho*	Zygadenus paniculatus
	Kogi a donup *P*	
	Kogi desme *W*	
	E cramps *Bft*	
Desert Beauty	Ma good te hupi *P*	Dalea spp.
	Tsoho-mozick *W*	
Desert Mallow	Muha *P*	Sphaeralcea ambigua
	Numanaka *Elko Sho*	
	Koopena *Moapa P*	
Desert Rue; Turpentine-Broom	Mogurup	Thamnosma montana
Desert Star	See kope (Gum Plant) *Sho*	Stephanomeria exigua
	Waaha nane *W*	
Desert Trumpet	Tosanan bawkip *DVSho*	Eriogonum inflatum
	Baba gorum *Moapa P*	
Devil Horn; Unicorn Plant	E hook *Papago*	Proboscidea louisianica
	Muzza tacion *DVSho*	
Dock	Pawia *P*	Rumex crispus
	Modup *W*	
	Woosia *Elko Sho*	
Dodder		Cuscuta spp.
Dogwood; Osier	Atsa wish tsi danabu (first baby basket tree) *P*	Cornus stolonifera
	Gwinjera *Sho*	
	Badosanich *W*	
	Lotzanee *WS* (2nd bark used in Kinni-kinnick)	
Elderberry, blue	Hubu *P*	Sambucus caerulea
	Mutha paho *WS* (wood)	
	Muth'p *WS* (berries)	
Elderberry, red	Koono gibu *P*	Sambucus microbotrys
	Du hiem buh *S*	
Elk Lily; Deer Tongue; Green Gentian; Turret Lily		Frasera speciosa
Evening Primrose, white	Mozippe	Oenothera spp.
Evening Primrose, yellow	Koatsa dabe buha *P*	Oenothera hookeri
	Toya notz worda *Ft. Hall Sho*	
Eye medicine, Spurge	Tubicai *Moapa P*	
False Hellebore	Tobassop	Veratrum californicum
	Wundavassop *Sho*	
	Baduppa *W*	
	Butiwe *P*	

COMMON NAME	INDIAN NAME	BOTANICAL NAME
False Lupine; see Golden Pea		
Fiddleneck, white; see Chinese Pusley		
Flax, blue	Poohi natesua *Sho*	Linum lewisii
	Alai natesua *P*	
Four-o'clock	Hewovey *P*	Mirabilis bigelovii
	Dybaw *Sho*	var. retrorsa
	Panisamobe *Sho*	
Fungus	Apo pik a tiss *Bft*	Polyporus
Fungus; Punk on Douglas Fir	Nookt-nookt *Wasco, Ore.*	Fomes laricus
	Shuppenchush *WS*	
	Coonch (roasted & ground)	
Garlic	Padzimo *Sho*	Allium falcifolium
Gilia	Aqui he binga *Sho*	Gilia spp.
Gilia, blue	Tsai yarrabuh *P*	
Ginger, wild	Winnotme	Asarum caudatum
	Tukawatut *WS*	
Golden Pea; Golden Banner	So wee wee *P*	Thermopsis gracilis
Gooseberry	Mogoonsium	Ribes spp.
Gourd, Buffalo; Melon, Wild	Arnoko *Moapa P*	Cucurbita foetidissima
	Poonono *Sho*	
Grass, Basket; see Bear Grass		
Grass, Big; Sugar Cane	Mogoko *P*	Phragmites communis var. berlandieri
Grass, Bunch	Sopeeva *P L P*	
Grass, short	Buip *Sho*	
Grass, Sweet; see Sweet Grass		
Greasewood	Tonobe *P & Sho*	
Ground Cherries	Sat a upe	
Gum Plant	Aks peis *Bft*	Grindelia squarrosa
	Sanaka para *Sho*	
	Ithi wa hyine *Arapaho*	
Gum Plant	See kope, Samoko *Sho*	Stephanomeria exigua
	Wahanane *W*	Lygodesmia spinosa
Hawthorn	Ash num ma sho *WS*	Crataegus columbiana
	Simnasho *WS*	
	Wenapish *Bnk*	
Honeysuckle		Lonicera interrupta
Horehound; Soldier Tea		Marrubium vulgare
Horsetail; Joint Grass	Mep *W*	Equisetum arvense
Huckleberry	We woono wash *WS*	Vaccinium spp.
Indian Balsam	Toza *P & Sho*	Lomatium dissectum
	Doza *W*	var. multifidum
	Cha luksh *WS*	
	Neet a tat *Arapaho*	
	O muck kas *Bft*	
Indian Cabbage; Prince's Plume		Stanleya pinnata
Indian Hemp; Dogbane; see Milkweed	Weha, Wisha, Wana *Sho*	Apocynum & Asclepias spp.
Indian Onion	Saukipi satsi nikim *Bft*	Allium spp.

—67—

COMMON NAME	INDIAN NAME	BOTANICAL NAME
Indian Onion, white fl.	Show mo mee *WS*	
	Sham am way *WS*	
Indian Onion, pink fl.	Bostick *W*	
Indian Onion, 1 stem	Ammo, Gunk *Sho*	
Indian Onion, more than 1 stem	Ginga *Sho*	
Indian Paintbrush	Dosh mooye hanguna *P*	Castilleja spp.
	Taqua winnop	
	Doo wan dayem *Sho*	
Indian Potatoes; see Sand Food		
Indian Rhubarb; Cow Parsnip	Po kintsomo *Bft*	Heracleum lanatum
Indian Rice Grass; Sand Grass	Wye *P & S*	Oryzopsis hymenoides
Indian Rouge		Plagiobothrys fulvus var. campestris
Indian Tea; see Mormon Tea		
Indian Tobacco	Pwui bamo (green) *Sho*	Nicotiana spp.
	Bahombe (cured) *Sho*	
	Sawawa koop *Ute*	
	Sawak wape Moapa *P*	
Indian Turnip	Mass	Lithospermum linearifolium
Iris	Poku erop *P*	Iris missouriensis
	Daw see doya *Sho*	
	Pah sa gida *Sho*	
Jimson Weed; Stramonium	Moip *S*	Datura meteloides
	Tolache *Moapa P*	
Joshua Tree	Oomph *Sho*	Yucca brevifolia
	Tso-warm-up *Moapa P*	
Joshua Tree (fruits)	Ooss *Moapa P*	
Juniper	Wapi *P*	Juniper spp.
	Sammabe *Sho*	
	Poosh *WS*	
	Tsekie sino kosa *Bft*	
Juniper Berries	Sammapo *Sho*	
	Pawaap *Moapa P*	
Juniper, prickly	Bat they naw *Arapaho*	Juniperus communis var. saxatilis
Juniper, sweet fruited	Wapi-pui *P Owyhee*	
Krameria; Crimson Beak	Pahaab *Moapa P*	Krameria spp.
Larkspur	Multiko *DVSho*	Delphinium spp.
	D'lum d'lum *WS*	
Larkspur, red		Delphinium nudicaule
Licorice Root	Quitchemboo *Bnk*	Glycyrrhiza lepidota
Lily, Little Alpine	See lat aho *W*	Lilium parvum
Lily, Tiger	Tawho *Algonquin*	Lilium pardalinum
Lobelia		Lobelia cardinalis spp. graminea
Loco	Wa push me xtun *WS*	Astragalus spp.
Loco, inflated pod	Geputch (refers to cow poisoning)	Astragalus spp.
Loco, Rattleweed	A setse kutoko *Bft*	Astragalus spp.

COMMON NAME	INDIAN NAME	BOTANICAL NAME
Loco, slender pod	Gupushem *Sho*	
Loco, woolly	Tada ginobu *P*	Astragalus utahensis
Lupines, all	Wapeayta *WS*	Lupinus spp.
Lupine, Silver	Dellem *W*	
	Gopusimbe *Sho*	
	Cupi chuk *Sho*	
	Kamo sigi *P*	
Madder		Galium boreale
Meadow Rue	Esteewia *WS*	Thalictrum spp.
	Taba emul *W*	
	Pawaga *Sho*	
Melon, Wild; see		
Gourd, Buffalo		
Mesquite	Pemp *Moapa P* (bows)	Prosopis spp.
Mesquite, Honey	Ah pee (food)	Prosopis juliflora
		var. torreyana
Mesquite, Screw Bean	Qui erra (food)	Prosopis pubescens
Milkweed	Banumb (for horse's back)	Asclepias cryptoceras
Milkweed, big	Bija wavoko *Sho*	Asclepias speciosa
	Kosewich *Sho*	
	Wipanabu *P*	
	Se-talcht *Ore, Yakima*?	
Milkweed, Mexican		Asclepias fascicularis
Mimulus; Monkey Flower;	Unda vich quana *Sho*	Mimulus guttatus
Roper's Relief	Pah what na abe *P*	
Mormon Tea; Brigham;	Durumbe *Sho*	Ephedra spp.
Joint Fir	Tsurupe *P*	
	Tu tumbe *DVSho*	
	Tu tupe Moapa *P*	
Moss, Black	Wa kam wa *WS*	Alectoria fremontii
Moss, Yellow	Wapi-tonega *P*	
	Yugar sanibe *Sho*	
Mountain	Toyabe *Sho*	
Mountain, little	Dooya toyabe *Sho*	
Mountain, snow	Dakka toyabe *Sho*	
Mountain Balm;	Moon-num Moon-num *WS*	Ceanothus velutinus
Snow Brush;	Datzip *Sho*	
Squaw Tea;		
Sheep Herder Tea		
Mountain Balm No. 2;		Eriodictyon
Yerba Santa		californicum
Mountain Mahogany	Toobe *P*	Cercocarpus ledefolius
	Durumbe *Sho*	
	Dunumbe *Moapa P*	
	Turumbe *SkVSho*	
	Duhul (bark)	
Mountain Mahogany,		Cercocarpus betuloides
from California		
Muhly; Packsaddle Grass;	Winnets sonib *P*	Muhlenbergia squarrosa
Salt Ground Grass	Ona wahabe *P*	
Mule Ears; Sunflower	Wodzi kuh P	Wyethia mollis
Mustard;	Boina *Sho*	Cruciferae
Old Maid Sister;	Etsa *P*	
Not Much Seed;	Hama *Pyramid Lake P*	
Jim Hill Mustard	Metsum *W*	Descaurainia spp.

COMMON NAME	INDIAN NAME	BOTANICAL NAME
Nut Grass; Grass Nut	Taboose *P*	Cyperus rotundus
Oak, Gambel	Tsonips (tree), Cupmish "Cuppen" root diggers made from it. Wa wachee (acorns) all *WS*	
Onions; see Indian Onion		
Orchid; Pine Cone	Ane *Pyramid Lake P*	
Oregon Grape	O ti toque *Bft* Kawdanup *P* Sogo tiembuh *Sho* Ch' cow cow *WS*	Berberis repens
Osage Orange; Bow-wood	Boise d'arc, Bodark (French for bow-wood)	Maclura aurantiaca
Paint	Oapi (before cooking) *Sho* Bishapi (after cooking)	
Paint, not red	Buzup	
Paint, rock	Odumbe *P & Sho*	
Paint, white clay	Ee-bee *P & Sho*	
Paintbrush, red; see Indian Paintbrush		
Paintbrush, yellow	E si match sis *Bft*	Orthocarpus luteus
Pasque Flower	Napi *Bft*	Anemone occidentalis
Pemmican	Makakin *Bft* Wasna *Sioux*	
Pennyroyal, big	Guy mohpu *Sho*	Monarda spp.
Pennyroyal, little		Mentha arvensis
Penstemon, small flower	Tu pasi wup we *P* Yah a te sa *P*	Penstemon breviflorus
Penstemon, white	Dimbashego *Sho*	Penstemon deustus
Peony, wild	Doo yah gum hoo *W* Tue ago nemo *W* Batipi *NP* Newatama *P* Olap cut olapcut *Nez Perce*	Paeonia brownii
Peppermint	Kush stick *WS* Cax si simmo *Bft* Paquanah *P & Sho*	Mentha piperita
Pepperwood; California Bay		Umbellularia californica
Phlox, pink; Stansbury Phlox	Saga donzia	Phlox longifolia
Phlox, Trumpet	Tem paiute *P & Sho* Paga gibe *P*	Ipomopsis aggregata
Pine Drops		Pterospora andromedea
Pine Nut	Tuba *P* Wapi *Sho*	
Pink Plumes	So yaits *Bft* Pa wa rabish *P*	Geum ciliatum
Pink Root	(Arapaho medicine)	Ivesia gordonii
Plantain	Woodie *SmVSho*	Plantago major
Plums, dried, pitted	Tuyu *NP*	
Poison Hemlock	Hakinop *P & Sho*	Cicuta douglasii
Poison Parsnip; Water Hemlock	A lem milla *WS*	
Poppy, California		Eschscholzia californica

COMMON NAME	INDIAN NAME	BOTANICAL NAME
Poverty Weed	Durunzip *Sho*	Iva axillaris
Primrose; see Evening Primrose		
Queen Anne's Lace; or	Eppaws *NP*	Perideridia gairdneri
Trail Potato	Yomba, Sowettuk *WS*	
Quinine Bush	Doomaya *Sho* (refers to kinni-kinnick mixture)	Garrya elliptica
Rabbit Brush, gray	Baw buh *W*	Chrysothamnus nauseosus
	Samoko *Sho*	
	Ange tabishapi *Sho*	
Rabbit Brush, green	Seebape (gum) *Sho*	Chrysothamnus spp.
Rabbit Guts	Kumi segee *P*	Glyptopleura marginata
Ramona; Little Chia	Tube sigino	Salvia dorrii
Redbud	Millay *Pomo*	Cercis occidentalis
Rye Grass	Washo *W* (tribe named for this)	Elymus condensatus
	Waiya, Bia sonib *Sho*	
Rye Grass, blades	Po hekawa hane *P*	
Sage, bud	Bombe *Sho*	Artemisia spinescens
	Kube *P*	
Sage, Mt. Ball	Kaksamis *Bft*	Artemisia frigida
Sage, white	Sissop *P*	Eurotia lanata
	Kosi wayab *Sho*	
Sagebrush, big	Sawabe *P* & *Sho*	Artemisia tridentata
	Sawak *Moapa P*	
Sagebrush, black	Bahabe *SmVSho*	Artemisia nova
Sagebrush, seed	Dabel *W*	
Sagebrush, small	Pava hobe	Artemisia ludoviciana
	Kose wiup	
Sagebrush, sweet; or	Pawots *Sho*	Artemisia dracunculus
False Tarragon	K'Tonee *WS*	
Salt Plant; Sweet Coltsfoot		Petasites palmata
Sand Dock	Tuha konobe *Sho*	Rumex hymenosepalus
	Tua ono gibu *P*	
	Ha-ne-sae-huit *Arapaho*	
Sand Food	Unh *Sho*	Ammobroma sonorae
Sand Grass; Indian	Wye *P* & *Sho*	Oryzopsis hymenoides
Rice Grass	Sum sut *W*	
Sand Verbena	Ayaho	Abronia latifolia
Sandalwood, lost blue		Comandra pallida
Sandwort	(used in kinni-kinnick)	Arenaria spp.
Screw Bean	Mesqueroo, Tornillo, Quierem all *Moapa P*	
Sea Holly	Momonu kaiyu *P*	Eryngium alismaefolium
Sedge, Nebraska		Carex nebrascensis
Sego Lily; Mariposa Lily	Kokse *W*	Calochortus nuttallii
	Kogi *P*	(Utah state flower)
	Segaw *Sho*	
	Noona *Ore*	
Service Berry;	Tuambe, Tuyembee *Sho*	Amelanchier pallida
Sarvis Berry	Kahso *WS*	
	Ok a nook *Bft*	
	Saskatoon *BC*	

COMMON NAME	INDIAN NAME	BOTANICAL NAME
Signal Plant; see Cliff Rose		
Silver Berry; Buffalo Berries	Cupsi (berries) *Bft*	Shepherdia argentea
Sneezeweed		Helenium hoopesii
Snowberry	Pambigama *P*	Symphoricarpos acutus
	Newa *Sho*	
Soaproot	Amole	Chlorogalum pomeridianum
Solomon's Seal; Fat Solomon	Shapui *P* Roy *Sho*	Smilacina racemosa var. amplexicaulis
Solomon's Seal; Slim Solomon; Thin Solomon	Add-at-a-pel *W* Wambona *Sho* Than-suv *Moapa P*	Smilacina stellata
Spearmint	Yam baguana *P* Bawana *Sho*	Mentha spicata
Spurge; see Eye Medicine		
Squaw Bush; see Sumac		
Stone Seed; Western Gromwell; Columbia Puccoon	Nemesaw Notmisha *Sho*	Lithospermum rederale
String Plant; see Licorice Root	Pooy sonib *P*	Psoralea lanceolata
String Plant; Leather Root (California)		Psoralea macrostachya
Sugar Cane; Indian Taffy	Behabe *P* Pahrump Mogoko *P & Moapa P*	Phragmites communis var. berlandieri
Sulphur Flower	Naka donup *P*	Eriogonum umbellatum
Sumac; Squawbush Also called Lemonade Bush and Sugar Bush	See a wimb *Sho* Ish *Ute*	Rhus trilobata var. anisophylla
Sunflower; Balsam Root; Arrow-leaved (gray one) (green one) (large white one)	Ah Kerh *Sho* Sugilatse *W* Po' a' kerh Pava ah' kerh *P*	Balsamorhiza sagittata
Sunflower, big woolly	Kosi a guh *P*	Wyethia mollis
Sunflower, Prairie (poor one)	Pa-ak *P & Sho*	Helianthus petiolaris
Sweet Anise	Bossowey *Sho*	Osmorrhiza occidentalis
Sweet Cicely	Pach-co-i-au-saukas *Bft*	
Sweet Grass; Vanilla Grass	Se padzimo *Bft*	Hierochloe odorata
Tansy	Not native	Tanacetum vulgare
Tarweed; see vinegar weed		
Thistle	Koida *P* Thinna *Sho* Tzinga *Sho* Chia wugu *Moapa P*	Cirsium edule
Thistle Poppy	Tsagida *Sho* Ishub goofwa *P*	Argemone munita
Tobacco; see Indian Tobacco		
Toothache Plant; see Turtle Back		

COMMON NAME	INDIAN NAME	BOTANICAL NAME
Trail Potato; see Queen Anne's Lace		
Trumpet Phlox	Tem paiute *P & Sho*	Ipomopsis aggregata
Tule		Scirpus acutus
Turkey Mullein		Eremocarpus setigerus
Turtle Back	Sebu mogoonobu *Moapa P*	Psathyrotes ramosissima
Unicorn Plant; see Devil Horn		
Valerian	Gweeya *Sho*	Valeriana edulis
	Kuya *Northern P*	
Vinegar weed		Trichostema lanceolatum
Virgin's Bower; see Clematis		
Wheat Grass, slender	Sunu *P*	Agropyron trachycaulum
Wickiups; Round Houses	Kani *P*	
Wild Buckwheat	Naka-donup *all*	Eriogonum spp.
	Segwebee *Elko Sho*	
Wild Celery	Hobe *Sho*	Apium spp.
	Yeluts *P*	
	Mo-zook-addas *W*	
	Iknish *Klamath*	
	P-tish p-tish *WS*	
Wild Cucumber (California)		Marah fabaceus
Wild Currant; see Currant		
Wild Parsley		Sium suave
Wild Parsnip; see Poison Hemlock		
Wild Peach	Tsanavi *P*	Prunus andersonii
Wild Rose	Tsiavi *P & Sho*	Rosa spp.
	Pat sur malle *W*	
	Yano *Arapaho*	
	Tschapa *WS*	
Willow, all	Tsube *P & Sho*	Salix spp.
	Himmo *W* (arbors)	
Willow, Arroyo		Salix lasiolepis
Willow, Black		Salix nigra
Willow, broadleaf	Sagup *Sho*	
Willow, cradleboard	Kaga oop *Moapa*	
Willow, desert	Kanab *Moapa*	Chilopsis linearis
Willow, Gray; or Coyote Willow	Kosi tsube *Sho*	Salix argophylla
Willow; Silver, Valley or Sandbar		Salix hindsiana
Winter Fat; White Sage	Sissop *P & Sho*	Eurotia lanata
Wire Grass	Sineva, pondaseep *Sho*	Juncus balticus
Wolf Moss	Yugur sanibe, luke komo *Wasco*	Evernia vulpina
	Tama muklth muklth *WS*	
Woman medicine	Paguidobe *Moapa P*	Porophyllum (probably gracile)
Wormwood (California)	Poonkinny	Artemisia trifurcata

COMMON NAME	INDIAN NAME	BOTANICAL NAME
Yarrow	Pannonzia *Sho*	Achillea lanulosa
	Wiutu *P*	
	Kannam nam stuck *Wasco*	
	Wapun wapun *WS*	
Yellow Bell	Kana qut'l ch'k *Wasco*	Fritillaria pudica
	Stakhs *WS*	
Yerba Buena		Satureja douglasii
(California)		
Yerba Mansa	Ch'ponip *Moapa P*	Anemopsis californica
	Nupitchi *Sho*	
Yucca, small	Datil, Ooss *Moapa P*	Yucca baccata
Yucca, tall one	Viemp *Moapa P*	Yucca whipplei

INDEX OF SCIENTIFIC NAMES

Abies
  lasiocarpa, 37,57
Abronia
  villosa, 41
Acacia
  greggii, 57
  spp., 39
Acer
  spp., 5
Achillea
  lanulosa, 43,45,47,49
Adiantum
  jordani, 4
  pedatum
    aleuticum, 4,5
Aesculus
  californica, 5,17,25,55
Alectoria
  fremontii, 17
Allium
  falcifolium, 14,33
Alnus
  spp., 4,10,14
Amaranthus
  graecizans, 32
Amelanchier
  alnifolia, 2,22
  pallida, 2,22
  spp., 53
Ammobroma
  sonorae, 16
Anemone
  occidentalis, 43
Anemopsis
  californica, 38,46
Angelica
  breweri, 50
Apium
  spp., 23,29,45,57
Apocynum
  cannabinum, 60
  spp., 10,52
Arctostaphylos
  uva-ursi, 61
Arenaria
  congesta, 42,47
  spp., 39,61
Argemone
  hispida, 42,44
  platyceras
    hispida, 42,44
Artemesia
  arbuscula
    nova, 42

douglasiana, 40,43
dracunculoides, 29,51
dracunculus, 29,51
frigida, 38,51,54
gnaphalodes, 46,51
heterophylla, 40,43
ludoviciana, 46,51
spinescens, 41
tridentata, 44,51,54
spp., 10,17,42,55
Asclepias
  cryptoceras, 49
  fascicularis, 47
  mexicana, 47
  speciosa, 56
  spp., 10,60
Astragalus
  purshii
    lagopinus, 38
  spp. 29
Balsamorhiza
  sagittata, 23,26,51,56
Berberis
  repens, 42,45
  spp., 10,44
Betula
  spp., 14
Brassica
  spp., 23
Brodiaea
  spp., 13
Calocedrus
  decurrens,
    2,10,24,52,56
Calochortus
  macrocarpus, 15
  nuttallii, 15
  spp., 13
Camassia
  quamash, 14
  spp., 13,14,15
Carex
  exsiccata, 8
  mendocinensis, 6
  nebraskensis, 51
Carum
  gairdneri, 16,33
Castilleja
  spp., 50
Ceanothus
  velutinus, 40
  spp., 57
Cercis
  occidentalis, 3,5,6

Cercocarpus
  betuloides, 52,62
  ledefolius, 38,51,52,53,
    54
Chaenactis
  stevioides, 40
Chenopodium
  album, 23
Chilopsis
  linearis, 52
Chimaphila
  umbellata
    occidentalis, 61
Chlordgalum
  pomeridianum, 20,57
Chrysothamnus
  nauseosus, 54
  spp., 42,56
Claytonia
  perfoliata, 23
Clematis
  ligusticifolia, 40,47,52,
    57,59
  spp., 49
Cleome
  serrulata, 40,53
Cogswellia
  cous, 12
  spp., 57
Coldenia
  spp., 16
Comandra
  pallida, 53,59
Conium
  maculatum, 47
Corallorhiza
  maculata, 37
Cornus
  occidentalis, 5
  stolonifera, 2,10,40
  spp., 20,61
Corylus
  californica, 6,25
Covillea
  tridentata, 37,45,47,52
Crataegus
  columbiana, 22
Curcurbita
  foetidissima, 47,48,50
Cuscuta
  spp., 54
Cyperus
  rotundus, 16

Dalea
spp., 38,43,51
Datura
meteloides, 48,50
Delphinium
nudicaule, 50
Echinocystis
spp., 41
Echinodontia
tinctoria, 54
Eleagnus
argentea, 21,56
Elymus
condensatus, 17
Ephedra
spp., 47
Epicampes
rigens, 8
Equisetum
arvense, 44,57
spp., 51
Eremocarpus
setigerus, 20,21
Erigeron
concinnus, 47
pumilus
concinnoides, 47
Eriodictyon
californicum, 38
Eriogonum
inflatum, 62
umbellatum, 37
spp., 17
Eryngium
alismaefolium, 42
Eschscholzia
californica, 45
Euphorbia
arenicola, 39
occellata
arenicola, 39
Eurotia
lanata, 17
Evernia
vulpina, 4,44,53,54
Fomes
laricus, 54,55
Galium
boreale, 54
tinctorum, 54
trifidum
subbiflorum, 54
triflorum, 57
spp., 10,53,54
Garrya
elliptica, 61

Geum
ciliatum, 39,57
Gilia
aggregata, 42,48,53
spp., 37,56
Glycyrrhiza,
lepidota, 38
Glyptopleura,
marginata, 23
Grindelia
squarrosa, 37
serrulata, 43,45
Gutierrezia
sarothrae, 54
Helenium
hoopesii, 38
Heliotropium
curassavicum
oculatum, 41
Heracleum
lanatum, 23,50
Hesperonia
retrorsa, 44,46,57
Heuchera
glabella, 39,49,53
parvifolia, 39,43
spp., 43
Hierochloe
odorata, 51
Horkelia
gordonii, 40
Ipomopsis
aggregata, 42,48,53,56
Iris
douglasiana, 60
missouriensis, 41,45
spp., 47
Iva
axillaris, 42
Ivesia
gordonii, 40
Juncus
mexicanus, 8
Juniperus
communis
saxatilis, 50
scopulorum, 50
siberica, 50
utahensis, 41
spp., 10,19,26,43,46,
47,50,52,53,55,56
Larrea
tridentata, 37,45,47,52
Lepargyraea
argentea, 32
canadensis, 17,21

Leptotaenia
multifida, 23,37,39,49,
55
Lewisia
rediviva, 12,13,38
Libocedrus
decurrens, 2,10,24,52,
56
Linum
lewisii, 39,44
Lithocarpus
densiflora, 24
Lithospermum
linearifolium, 50
ruderale, 42,46
spp., 50,54
Lomatium
cous, 12
dissectum var.
multifidum, 23,37,
39,47,49,55
spp., 57
Lonicera
interrupta, 5,44
Lycium
spp., 21
Lygodesmia
spp., 56
Maclura
aurantiaca, 52
Mammillaria
microcarpa, 23
Marah
spp., 41
Martynia
proboscides, 7
Mentha
arvensis, 41
penardi, 45
piperita, 45
rotundifolia, 38
Mentzelia
albicaulis, 27
spp., 32
Mimulus
guttatus, 43
Mirabilis
bigelovii var.
retrorsa, 44,46,57
Monarda (?)
spp., 38
Monardella
odoratissima, 45
Montia
perfoliata, 23

Muhlenbergia
  rigens, 8
Nicotiana
  spp., 4,5,60,61,62
Nolina
  bigelovii, 9
Nuphar
  polysepalum, 29
Oenothera
  caespitosa, 44
  hookeri, 50
Opuntia
  engelmannii, 22
  occidentalis, 22
  spp., 17,46
Orthocarpus
  luteus, 54
Oryzopsis
  hymenoides, 26,27,32
Osmorhiza
  occidentalis, 29,38,41,
  49
Pachylophis
  caespitosus, 44
Paeonia
  brownii, 38
Parmelia
  molluscula, 53
Parosela
  spp., 38,43,50,51
Penstemon
  breviflorus, 44
  deustus, 44,47
  spp., 42
Perideridia
  gairdneri, 16,33
Petasites
  palmatus, 25
Philadelphus
  lewisii
    gordonianus, 52
  spp., 51
Phlox
  longifolia, 44
Phoradendron
  californicum, 63
Phragmites
  communis
    berlandieri, 52
Physaria
  didymocarpa, 38
Picea
  spp., 2,4
Pinus
  edulis, 44
  monophylla, 25

sabiniana, 2,5,6,25
  spp., 9,19,54,56
Plagiobothrys
  campestris, 55
  fulvus
    campestris, 55
Plantago
  major, 43
Populus
  tremuloides, 17
  spp., 17,54
Porophyllum
  leucospermum, 46
  spp., 46
Potentilla
  spp., 42
Proboscidea
  louisianica, 7,9,10
Prosopis
  juliflora
    torreyana, 27,52,56
  pubescens, 27
Prunus
  andersonii, 38
  virginiana
    demissa, 21,32,42
    melanocarpa, 21,54
  spp., 54
Pseudotsuga
  menziesii, 5,6
Psathyrotes
  ramosissima, 39,41,45
Psoralea
  esculenta, 13
  lanceolata, 38,59
  macrostachya, 59
Pterospora
  andromedea, 49
Pulsatilla
  occidentalis, 43
Purshia
  tridentata, 50,53
  spp., 43,45,56
Quercus
  garryana, 24
  kelloggii, 24
  spp., 6,10,18,24,54
Ramona
  incana, 38
Ratibida
  columnaris, 54
Rhamnus
  purshiana, 42
Rhus
  diversiloba, 6,56
  trilobata, 17,53,54
  spp., 60

Ribes
  aureum, 22,43
  cereum, 22,50
  petiolare, 22
  spp., 32
Robinia
  pseudo-acacia, 55
Rosa
  nutkana, 22
  spauldingii, 22
  spp., 3,17,38,43,54
Rumex
  crispus, 43,49
  hymensepalus, 44
  venosus, 42,54
Sagittaria
  latifolia, 13
Salix
  exigua, 42
  hindsiana, 2,3
  lasiandra, 7
  lasiolepis, 60
  spp.,
  6,10,28,32,52,57,58,59
Salvia
  Columbariae, 28
  Dorrii, 38
Sambucus
  caerulea, 22,42,57
  glauca, 22,42,57
  microbotrys, 22
  racemosa, 22
  spp., 57
Satureja
  douglasii, 17
Savastana
  odorata, 51
Scirpus
  fluviatilis, 6
  maritimus, 6
  spp., 57
Scrophularia
  spp., 17,53
Shepherdia
  argentea, 21,32,56
  canadensis, 17,21
Sieversia
  ciliata, 39,57
Smilacina
  racemosa
    amplexicaulis, 46
  stellata, 39
Sphaeralcea
  ambigua, 43,46,56
Stanleya
  pinnata, 23

—77—

Symphoricarpos
  racemosus, 52
  rivularis, 52
Tanacetum
  crispum
    vulgare, 46
  vulgare, 46
Taxus
  brevifolia, 51
Tetradymia
  glabrata, 56
Thalictrum
  spp., 37,48,57
Torreya
  californica, 6,56
Trichostema
  lanceolatum, 20,21
Trifolium
  fucatum
    virescens, 23
  virescens, 23

Tumion
  californica, 6
Typha
  latifolia, 23,55
  spp., 10
Umbellularia
  californica, 25,43
Usnea
  lacunosa, 55
Vaccinium
  spp., 10,18
Valeriana
  dioica
    sylvatica, 45
  edulis, 16
  septentrionalis, 45
Veratrum
  californicum, 45,46,47
  speciosum, 62
  spp., 49
Viola
  spp., 10

Vitis
  spp., 5,6
Washingtonia
  (see Ozmorhiza)
  divaricata, 49
Woodwardia
  fimbriata, 4
  radicans, 4
Wyethia
  longicaulis, 43
Xerophyllum
  tenax, 2,4,5
Yucca
  baccata, 57
  brevifolia, 8,10
  glauca, 57
  spp., 10
Zigadenus
  paniculatus, 45
  spp., 42

INDEX OF COMMON NAMES

Acacia, 39
Alder, 4,10,14
Alfalfa, 59
Alkali Lily, 44
Alum Root, 39,43,49,53
Angelica, 50
Antelope Brush, 39,43, 45,47,50,53,56
Arrowhead, 13
Arrow wood, 51
Ash, 62
Aspen, 17
Aster, 42,47
Ballhead Sandwort, 42, 47
Balsamroot, 45
Bay, California, 25,43
Bear berry, 61
Bed Straw, 54,57
Bee plant, 17,40,53
Biscuit root, 12,13,57
Birch, 14
Bitter root, 13,38
Bladder Pod, 38
Blazing Star, 27
Blue Curls, 20,21
Breadroot, 13
Bride's Bouquet, 40
Brigham Tea, 47
Broadiaea, 13
Buckeye, 17,20,25
Buckberry, 21,32
Buckthorn, 57
Buck wheat, 17,37
Buffalo Berry, 17,21,32
Buffalo Gourd, 47
Bull Berry, 21
Bulrush, 42
Buttercup, 27
Cactus, 17,22,40
Cactus, Prickly Pear, 46
Camas Lily, 13,14,15,42
Camas, Death, 45
Carrot, wild, 55
Cascara, 42
Cats Claw, 57
Cat Tail, 10,23,55
Cedar, 2,10,50,52,56,59
Cedar, Incense, 24
Cedar brush, 56
Celery, wild, 23,29,45,57
Chestnut, 55
Chokecherry, 21,32,42, 54

Chia, 28,38
Cinquefoil, 42,54
Citrus plant, 51
Clematis, 40,47,49,52, 57,59
Cleome, 40,53
Clover, 23,25
Coffee Berry, 42
Coneflower, 54
Conk, 55
Coral Root, 37
Corn, 10,28,47,54
Cottonwood, 17
Cow Parsnip, 23
Creosote Bush, 37,45, 47,52
Creosote, mistletoe, 62
Cucumber, 41
Currant, 32,43
Currant, bear, 22,50
Currant, black, 22
Currant, golden, 22
Currant, wax, 22
Datura, 50
Desert Mallow, 43,46,56
Desert Gum, 56
Desert Rue, 51
Desert Trumpet, 62
Devil Horn, 7,9,10
Dock, 43,49
Dodder, 54
Dogwood, 2,5,10,20,40, 61
Elder, 57
Elderberry, 22,42,57
Elk Lily, 17
Ephedra, 47
Evening Primrose, 50
Evening Star, 27
False Maidenhair, 57
Fern, 6,23
Fern, Five Finger, 4,5
Fern, giant, 4
Fern, Maidenhair, 4
Fiddleneck, 41
Fir, 6
Fir, Balsam, 37,57
Fir, Douglas, 55
Fir, Joint, 17
Flax, blue, 39,44
Forget-me-not, white, 55
Four o'clock, 44,46,57
Garlic, 14
Gentian, 17

Geranium, 43,46,56
Giant Rye, 17
Gilia, 37
Golden Prince's Plume, 23
Golden Seal, 54
Goosefoot, 27
Gourd, 50
Grass, basket, 2,4,5,9
Grass, bear, 9
Grass, deer, 8
Grass, Indian Rice, 26
Grass, joint, 42,57
Grass, nut, 16
Grass, rye, 39
Grass, sand, 26,27,32
Grass, squaw, 10
Grass, sweet, 51
Grass, wild mountain, 32
Grass, wire, 8,17
Grapevine, 5,6
Ground Plum, 29
Gum Plant, 37,43,45
Haw Bush, 22
Hawthorn, black, 22
Hazel brush, 1,2,5,6,7
Hazel nut, 25
Hellebore, False, 45,46, 47,49
Hellebore, white, 62
Honey Mesquite, 27
Honeysuckle, 5,44
Horse Tail, 44,51,57
Huckleberry, 10,18
Impetigo Plant, 44
Indian Apple, 13
Indian Balsam, 23,37,39, 40,47,49,62
Indian Cabbage, 23
Indian Gravy, 27
Indian Hemp, 10,52,59
60
Indian Lettuce, 23
Indian Onion, 13
Indian Paint Brush, 50
Indian Potato, 13,33
Indian Rhubarb, 23,50
Indian Tea, 17,47
Indian Tobacco, 62
Indian Turnip, 13,50
Iris, 41,45,47,60
Jimson Weed, 48,50
Joshua Tree, 8,10

Juniper, 10,19,41,43,45, 46,47,50,52,53,55,56
Kuha, 32
Lady Finger, 23
Lambs Quarter, 23,27
Larkspur, red, 50
Leather root, 59
Lichen, ground, 53
Licorice root, 38
Lizard Tail, 46
Lobelia, 42
Locust, 55,56
Lupine, 41
Madder, 10,54
Maple, 5
Meadow Rue, 37,48,57
Melon, wild, 48
Mesquite, 52,56
Milkweed, 10,47,49,56, 59,60
Milkweed, Mexican, 47
Miner's Lettuce, 23
Mint, horse, 38
Mock Orange, 52
Monkey flower, 43
Morman Tea, 17,47
Moss, black, 17
Moss, gray, 55
Moss, Wolf, 4,44,53,54
Mountain Balm, 38,40
Mountain Mahogony, 13, 38,39,51,52,53,54,62
Mugwort, 51
Mustard, 23,28,32
Nicotiana, 60
Nutmeg, 6,56
Oak, 10,54
Oak, black, 24
Oak, tan, 24
Oak, white, 24,54
Onion, 14,33,35
Opuntia, 17
Oregon Grape, 10,42, 45,54
Osage Orange, 52,54
Paintbrush, yellow, 54
Parosela, 38,43,51
Parsnip, 47
Pasque Flower, 43
Peach, wild, 38
Peanut Butter Plant, 23
Pennyroyal, 29,41,45
Penstemon, 39,42,44,47
Peony, 38,39,49
Peppermint, 29,45
Pepperwood, 43

Peyote, 23
Phlox, Stansbury, 39,44
Phlox, Trumpet, 42,48, 53,56
Pine, 44,54,56,59
Pine, Digger, 2,5,6
Pine, Lodgepole, 58
Pine, Pinyon, 19,25,38, 53
Pine, Sweet, 57
Pine Drops, 49
Pink Plumes, 39,57
Pink Root, 40
Plantain, 43
Plant aux Perles, 46
Poison Oak, 6,56
Pond Lily, 29
Poplar, 54
Poppy, California, 45
Poverty Weed, 39,42
Prairie Apple, 13
Prickly Pear, 22
Primrose, 44
Prince's Pine, 61
Prince's Plume, 23
Queen Anne's Lace, 16
Quinine Bush, 61
Rabbit brush, 42,54,56
Rabbitguts, 23
Ramona, 38
Rattleweed, 38
Redbud, 1,5,6
Roper's Relief, 43
Rose, 17,22,38,43,54
Sage, 10,38,41,51
Sage, Black, 42
Sage, Mountain Ball, 38,51,54
Sage, Silver, 42
Sage, small, 42,46
Sage, white, 17
Sagebrush, 17,39,43,45, 51,54,55
Sand Dock, 42,44,54
Sand Potato, 16
Sand Verbena, 41
Sandalwood, 53,59
Sandwort, 39,61
Sarvis Berry, 22,53
Screw Bean, 27
Sea Holly, 42
Sedge, 6,8
Sedge, Nebraska, 51
Sego Lily, 15
Service Berry, 2,22,53
Shad Blow, 22

Silverberry, 56
Skunk Berry, 32
Sky Rocket, 48,53
Snakeweed, 54
Sneezeweed, 38
Snowberry, 52
Snowdrops, 55
Soap root, 20,57
Soloman's Seal, 46
Spearment, 29
Spruce, 2,4
Spurge, 39
Squaw Bush, 53
Squaw Root, 16
Starry Soloman's Seal, 39
Stone Seed, 42,46
String Plant, 38,59
Sugar Cane, wild, 52
Sumac, Golden, 60
Sumac, Three lobed, 17, 53,54
Sunflower, 17,23,26,43, 51
Sunflower, Balsam root, 26,56
Sweet Anise, 29,38,41
Sweet Cecily, 49
Sweet Coltsfoot, 25
Sweet Sage, 29
Syringa, 52
Tansy, 46
Tarweed, 29
Thistle Poppy, 42,44
Tobacco Root, 16
Trail Potato, 16,33
Tule, 13,58
Tule Mint, 41
Tule Potato, 13
Tumbleweed, 32
Turkey Mullein, 20,21
Turtleback, 39,41,45
Unicorn Plant, 7
Valerian, 16,45
Virgin's Bower, 57
Wild Caraway, 16
Wild Lilac, 57
Willow, 6,7,10,20,57, 58,59
Willow, Arroyo, 60
Willow, Desert, 52
Willow, Grey, 42
Willow, Silver, 2
Wolf Berry, 21
Wormwood, 40,43,46
Yarrow, 43,45,47,49

Yerba Buena, 17
Yerba del Pasmo, 46

Yerba Mansa, 38,46
Yerba Santa, 38
Yew, 51

Yucca, 9,10,57
Yuki Salt Plant, 25